I0837747

ISBN: 9798591479824

30-DAY DIET

for

SENIOR WOMEN

1200-CALORIE

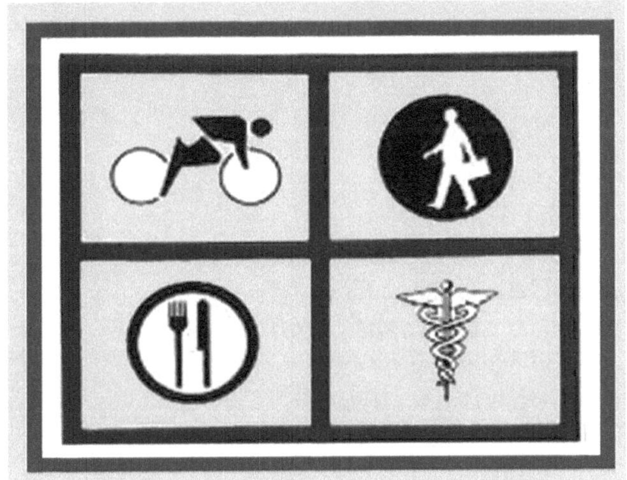

Vincent Antonetti, PhD
Tina Hudson, M.S.

NoPaperPress™

NOTE: At publication, the off-the-shelf foods used in portions of this book were widely available in most supermarkets. But food products come and go. So if there is a frozen entrée or soup selection in this diet that is out of stock, or that's been discontinued, or perhaps that you don't like, or that you forgot to pick up while shopping, please substitute another food that has **approximately** the same caloric value and nutritional content. In this regard, many dieters have found the foods listed in the Appendices at the end of this book to be very helpful.

CONTENTS

The Best Weight Loss Diets

According to the late Dr. Jean Mayer, of Tufts University's Department of Nutrition, a really good weight-loss diet must have the following three characteristics:

1) The diet must provide you with an understanding of weight control as well as the knowledge you need to reduce your weight to the desired level.

2) The diet must help you remain healthy while you are losing weight.

3) The diet must lead you to a healthier way of eating and exercising that

Why You Lose Weight

Most experts agree that when the energy value of the food you eat minus waste, equals the sum of your basal metabolic energy plus the energy you expend during physical activity, you will neither gain nor lose weight. They also agree that when you have an energy imbalance, you will either gain or lose weight. In general then:

- **Weight Maintenance** occurs when your food energy intake equals the total energy you expend in daily living. In this case your weight remains stable, i.e., you neither gain nor lose weight.

- **Weight Gain** occurs when your food energy intake is greater than the total energy you expend in daily living. In this case your body stores the extra energy as fat.

- **Weight Loss** occurs when your food energy intake is less than the total energy you expend in daily living. In this case your body converts stored fat (and in some cases muscle) into energy.

The measure of energy, whether in the form of food, physical activity, or heat, is the kilocalorie (hereafter simply called the Calorie). As already mentioned, weight loss occurs when you eat fewer calories than the calories you use in your day-to-day living. This difference in calories is referred to as your calorie deficit. How much weight you lose depends on the magnitude of your calorie deficit. (In technical terms, **the calorie deficit, or calorie difference, is the driving force for weight change**.)

Most people on a weight-loss diet want to know how much weight they will lose – and how fast. Simple metabolic calculations make a rough estimate possible. Physiologists have long known that to lose one pound requires a deficit of approximately 3500 Calories. Therefore, if a person's total calorie deficit over time is known, their weight loss over time can be calculated. (See "**Expected Weight Loss**" - page 8.) **In summary, if you eat and exercise such that you have a calorie deficit you will lose weight!**

Expected Weight Loss

On the *60-Day Diet - 1200 Calorie Edition*, <u>**most senior women lose 16 to 24 pounds.**</u> Smaller women, older women and less active women lose a bit less and larger women, younger women and more active women often lose more.

Exactly how much weight you will lose depends on how much you weigh, your age and your activity level. For the full story see *Weight Control - U.S. Edition* by Vincent W. Antonetti, Ph.D., an eBook also published by NoPaperPress.

First a Medical Exam

Everyone should at the very least have a medical assessment, or exam, before starting a weight loss diet. Why? You need to make sure your health will allow you to lower your caloric intake and increase your physical activity. Depending on your age and state of health, the medical checkup may be as simple as a visit to a physician who is familiar with your medical history, or it may be a thorough physical exam. The physician conducting the medical exam should be made aware of and should approve the specific weight loss diet you're planning. Additionally, if you are going to engage in some sort of physical activity in conjunction with this diet and especially if you have been totally inactive, or if you have or suspect you have cardiovascular disease or other health problems, or if you are obese, or if you are 40 or older, before embarking on the physical fitness portion of your weight control program you should have a stress test supervised by a physician. Finally, your physician can tell you how much and what type of exercise is right for you, how much you
should weigh, and prescribe a realistic weight- loss goal.

Eat Smart

No single food can supply all the nutrients you need in the amounts you need. The most important factors in nutrition are variety, variety, variety! **Variety is the key to a nutritious diet.** As a means of setting strategies for food selection, the U.S. Department of Health and Human Services and the Department of Agriculture issue

Dietary Guidelines every five years. The latest Dietary Guidelines describe a healthy diet as one that:
- Emphasizes fruits, vegetables, whole grains, and fat-free or low-fat milk products.
- Includes fish, poultry, lean meats, beans and nuts.
- Is low in saturated fats, trans fats, cholesterol, salt (sodium) and added sugars.
The latest guidelines encourage adults to consume a variety of nutrient-dense foods and beverages within their caloric needs. The afore mentioned U.S. government agencies recommend how much should be eaten from each of the basic food groups (i.e., from the fruit group, vegetable group, grains group, meat and beans group, dairy group, and oils group) to meet your caloric goal – whether you are trying to lose weight or maintain weight. All this information and more can be found in *Eat Smart - U.S. Edition* an eBook published by NoPaperPress.

Even though most adults can get all the vitamins and minerals they need by merely consuming a variety of nutritious foods (from the fruit group, the vegetable group, the grains group, the meat and beans group, the milk group, and the oils group), many physicians recommend a daily multi-vitamin/mineral supplement – just in case you don't eat the way you should.

Be aware that some micronutrients, such as the fat-soluble vitamin A, can be harmful if taken in large quantities. To be safe your multi-vitamin/mineral supplement should contain no more than 100 percent of the recommended dietary allowance (RDA) for each vitamin or mineral. Generally, you don't need the high doses in multi-vitamin/mineral supplements labeled "therapeutic" or "extra-strength." There may be medical reasons for taking larger amounts of a vitamin or mineral than the RDA provides, but check with your doctor first.

Tossed Salad

One of the dinner mainstays in the *60-Day Diet* is a "Tossed Salad." To prepare your "Tossed Salad" start with a bowl that has a volume of <u>at least</u> 16 ounces, or 2 cups. First add about 1 cup of either green leaf lettuce, Romaine lettuce or a Mesclun mix. Then add at least a half cup of other veggies such as broccoli, celery, cucumber, spinach, or watercress. This combination will total about 35 Calories

You'll be eating a "Tossed Salad" just about every day at dinnertime. Remember that variety is the key to a nutritious diet. So be sure to vary the ingredients of the salad. Top your Tossed Salad with 1½ tablespoons of any light salad dressing available at your local supermarket that contains no more than 25 Calories per tablespoon. Some of our favorites are:
- **Ken's Steakhouse Fat Free Raspberry Pecan**
- **Kraft Light Done Right House Italian**
- **Newman's Lighten Up! Balsamic Vinaigrette**
- **Wishbone Just 2 Good Honey Dijon**
Your "Tossed Salad" with salad dressing will cost you roughly 70 Calories but will be packed with lots of health-giving vitamins, minerals and fiber.

Regarding Bread

First understand that bread, more specifically whole-grain breads, are good sources of complex carbohydrates and dietary fiber, as well as the B vitamins (thiamin, riboflavin, niacin, and folate), vitamin E, and minerals (iron, magnesium and selenium). In recent years, however, sliced bread loaves have gotten larger, as have the bread slices inside these loaves. Just a few years ago the standard slice of bread contained about 65 to 70 Calories – now most are 100 plus Calories.

The 60-*Day Diet* requires whole-grain bread at 70 Calories per slice. Quite a few bakers sell thin sliced or "light" sliced bread. The difficult part is finding a whole grain thin sliced or "light" bread (with about 70 Calories per slice). Whatever the brand, make sure the first word in the Ingredients list is "whole." "Pepperidge Farm Small Slice 100% Whole Wheat" is a good choice. It's whole grain, has 70 Calories per slice and it tastes good too.

Substituting Foods

If there is a food listed in the *60-Day Diet* that you don't like, or perhaps that you forgot to pick up while shopping, you probably can exchange or substitute another food in its place – a technique used by dieticians. Exchanging a food listed in a diet for another food with approximately equal caloric value and nutritional content is the foundation of many successful long-term diets. Substitution possibilities are almost endless but have to be done carefully. The easiest substitutions are those within the same food group, such as exchanging one vegetable variety for another, or a glass of milk for a cup of yogurt. More sophisticated exchanges cross food groups, such as replacing 3½ ounces of turkey with a tablespoon of peanut butter on a piece of whole-wheat bread. Both foods are complete protein and both contain about 175 Calories. (Refer to a good online calorie table.) With some understanding and experience, you can use a calorie table to help you substitute foods called for in the *60-Day Diet* with equal calorie foods from the same food group.

Breakfast: You may substitute any cereal for any other wholesome cereal. For example, if you're not crazy about having Shredded Wheat for breakfast on Day 6, substitute Wheat Chex or Cheerios, etc. But remember to adjust the amount of cereal to account for the calorie difference between brands. If you don't like the soft-boiled egg called for on Day 9, cook a fried egg instead. And if Cantaloupe is on the menu but is not in season, replace cantaloupe with a half cup of orange juice – both contain about 50 Calories.

Snacks: Again, where 6 ounces of yogurt is specified you may substitute an 8-ounce glass of skim milk, but to maintain a nutritionally balanced diet keep this snack a dairy selection. Similarly, when fruit is on the agenda, you may select any type of fruit but do not stray from the fruit group. Nuts and popcorn can be interchanged at will. Specified convenient brand-name snacks, such as Skinny Cow ice cream, Kashi Granola bars, Nabisco 100 Calorie Pack cookies and Orville Redenbacher's Smart Pop Popcorn should be widely available but other equivalent brands may be substituted if need be. Just make sure the substitute snack has the same calorie count, or very close, to the specified snack.

Two Nights – No Cooking

Everyone deserves a break from the grind of preparing dinner after coming home from work. So the *60-Day Diet* gives you two days off per week! Notice that one night a week the meal plan calls for a frozen dinner and on a second night during the week you're encouraged to eat out. There are, however, some rules and caveats involved – these are covered in the next two sections.

Frozen Dinner Rules

In general, a frozen dinner should not be a meal in itself. Make sure you add a salad, fruit, bread etc. The frozen dinner you choose should come with at least one cup of cooked vegetables. If your frozen dinner doesn't measure up, add your own frozen, fresh or canned vegetables. And look for dinners with no more than 800 mg of sodium. In addition, make sure the dinner you choose has no more than 30 percent of the daily value for total fat. Appendix A on page 196 contains a comprehensive tabulation of reasonably good frozen dinner choices. And on the days when a frozen dinner is specified, you will be given a calorie goal for the frozen dinner. For example, Day 5 calls for frozen fish dinner with a maximum allowable 340 Calories. If you choose a frozen fish dinner that contains less than 340 Calories, you may spend the unused calories any way you wish.

Moreover, on those nights when you just don't have the energy or time to cook, you can always substitute a frozen dinner for the "Recipe of the Day" or the entree listed in the meal plan. For example, Day 2 calls for Herb-Crusted Cod for dinner. The total calorie count for dinner is 520. In place of the cod, any combination of a frozen fish dinner and side dishes (salads, etc) with a total calorie content close to 520 would be an acceptable, albeit not as tasty, alternative.

Eating Out Challenges

You may eat out once a week. When you're on a diet, however, eating in a restaurant can be a challenge, because most restaurant portions are huge, and can easily total more than 1000 Calories. On the *60-Day Diet*, a dinner type (i.e., fish, chicken, etc) and a calorie target is specified. For example Day 7 of the 1200 Calorie diet calls for a chicken dinner and allows you 530 Calories.

First, you need to choose a restaurant where you have a fighting chance to achieve your calorie goal. Next, order something simple, such as broiled fish with steamed vegetables and brown rice. Tell the waiter you want no sauce, no gravy, nothing added. Then, knowing your calorie objective, and that most fish and chicken are about 50 Calories per ounce, most steamed vegetable servings average approximately 50 Calories per cup, and rice is about 100 Calories per ½ cup, decide how much to eat and take the remainder home. If fresh fruit is not an option, pass on dessert and have the snack in the meal plan.

Important Notes

1) Coffee or tea may be caffeinated or decaf. If desired, skim milk and a sugar substitute may be added to coffee or tea, and **Soy or Almond** milk may be used instead of cow's milk.

2) Fried eggs or scrambled eggs should be cooked in a pan coated with a non-stick cooking spray. Hard-boiled eggs may be substituted for fried, scrambled or soft-boiled eggs.

3) Cereals should be whole grain and unsweetened. At the top of the list are Old-fashioned Oatmeal, Wheatena and Shredded Wheat. Among other reasonably healthy choices are Cheerios, Wheat Chex, Wheaties, some Kashi cereals and Farina. When blueberries are in season, you may **substitute blueberries for raisins** added to your cereal. (Approx. substitution ratio = 2 blueberries for one raisin.)

4) Bread may be either plain or toasted whole grain, such as whole wheat, whole rye or pumpernickel. Look for whole grain varieties that contain 70 Calories per slice. If desired, bread may be sprayed with a zero-calorie butter substitute.

5) When soup in a microwaveable bowl or a can is specified, eat only one serving (8 ounces) unless otherwise noted. (Microwaveable bowls and cans usually contain about two servings.)

6) Use freely as desired: clear unsweetened coffee, clear unsweetened tea, water, seltzer water and any diet soda, clear soups without fat, bouillon, and seasonings such as mustard, cinnamon, dill, herbs, red and black pepper, curry, vinegar, lemon juice and sections, and dill and sour pickles.

7) Use only lean cuts of meat trimmed of all visible fat. Poultry should be limited to chicken or turkey breasts (white meat only and skinless).

8) When canned tuna or salmon is specified, use fish **packed in water**.

9) When the diet calls for turkey bacon, make sure the brand you buy has no more than 35 Calories per slice.

10) An unlimited amount of green salad may be eaten, but the salad dressing should be as specified.

11) If it's more convenient, any food item may be moved to any part of the day and combined with any meal or snack.

12) If you cannot find the exact item called for in the diet (because it's out of stock or discontinued), substitute a comparable food (of the same type and close caloric value).

13) Take a daily **multi-vitamin/mineral supplement**. This is important when you're on a diet – as a kind of insurance policy.

Keeping It Off

Within five years, more than 90 percent of all dieters regain every pound they have lost. Why? In most cases it's because after losing weight most people eventually revert to their pre-diet eating and exercising habits,
and this inevitably leads to their regaining the weight they lost – and often more. Obviously after a diet you weigh less. The fact is the less you weigh, the less you need to eat to sustain your lower weight.

A study, published in the *Annals of Internal Medicine*, that followed 4,000 people for three decades suggests that in the long term, 90 percent of men and 70 percent of women will become overweight. Interestingly, half of the men and women in the study, who had made it well into adulthood without a weight problem, ultimately also became overweight and a third actually became obese. The point being that you can never
become complacent. You must continually watch your weight because we are all at risk of becoming overweight.

The key to long-term weight control success is knowledge and understanding, combined of course with desire and self-discipline. Once you reach your weight goal, I suggest you read ***Weight Maintenance - U.S. Edition*** by Vincent Antonetti, Ph.D. (also published by NoPaperPress) – considered the best weight maintenance eBook, or paperback, on the market.

1200 CALORIE DAILY MENUS

<h2 align="center">Day 1 Daily Menu</h2>

BREAKFAST	Calories	Totals
Grapefruit (½)	75	
Scrambled egg (See Notes - page 12)	80	
Whole grain toast (1 slice) (page 12)	70	
Coffee (page 12)	10	235 Cal
SNACK		
Coffee or tea	10	10 Cal
LUNCH		
Ham (2 oz) with mustard on 2 slices rye bread	290	
Pickle spear	0	
Hot or iced tea	10	300 Cal
SNACK		
Fresh fruit in season (apple, peach, etc)	70	
Coffee or tea	10	80 Cal
DINNER		
Chicken with Peppers & Onions (Recipe 1 page 46)	250	
Sautéed red peppers with onions (Recipe 1)	70	
Green beans (steamed) & mashed cauliflower	25	
Large tossed salad - 1½ Tbsp dressing (See page 10)	85	
Water with lemon wedge	15	475 Cal
SNACK		
Graham crackers (2 squares)	60	
Skim milk (4 oz = ½ cup)	45	105 Cal
		1205 Cal

<h1 style="text-align:center"><u>Day 2 Daily Menu</u></h1>

BREAKFAST	Calories	Totals
Orange juice (½ cup)	50	
Wheaties (¾ cup) + ½ cup skim milk + ½ banana	190	
Coffee	10	250
SNACK		
Fresh fruit in season (apple, pear, etc)	70	
Coffee or tea	10	80 Cal
LUNCH		
Soup (Appendix B - page 76)	110	
Turkey breast (1 oz) on 1 slice rye bread (½ sandwich)	105	
Pickle spear	0	
Lettuce & tomato slices	20	
Hot or iced tea	10	245
SNACK		
Coffee or tea	10	10 Cal
DINNER		
Baked Herb-Crusted Cod (Recipe 2 - page 47)	230	
Spinach (½ cup) steamed with garlic & drizzled	100	
Asparagus (8 spears cooked & drained)	25	
Baked potato (medium size) (No Butter!)	100	
Whole grain bread (1 slice)	70	
Water	0	525
SNACK		
Fiber One Chocolate Fudge Brownie	90	
Coffee or tea	10	100
		1210

Day 3 Daily Menu

BREAKFAST	Calories	Totals
Fresh or frozen strawberries (½ cup)	25	
French toasted English Muffin Recipe 3 - page 48	270	
Light syrup (1 Tbsp)	30	
Coffee	10	335 Cal
SNACK		
Coffee or tea	10	10 Cal
LUNCH		
Salad (3 oz can tuna, 1 tsp Evoo, onions, celery)	175	
Rye bread (1 slice)	70	
Small bunch of grapes	65	
Coffee or tea	10	320 Cal
SNACK		
Coffee or tea	10	10 Cal
DINNER		
Broiled veal chop (4 oz lean)	200	
Corn on the cob (1 medium ear) (No Butter!)	100	
Broccoli (½ cup steamed & drizzled with 1 tsp	70	
Large tossed salad - 1½ Tbsp dressing (See page 10)	85	
Fresh fruit in season (apple, peach, etc)	70	
Water	0	525 Cal
SNACK		
Coffee or tea	10	10 Cal
		1210 Cal

Day 4 Daily Menu

BREAKFAST	Calories	Totals
Grapefruit (½)	75	
Cheerios (1 cup) + ½ cup skim milk + 15 raisins*	190	
Coffee	10	275 Cal
SNACK		
Coffee or tea	10	10 Cal
LUNCH		
Cottage cheese (1 cup low fat)	180	
Large tossed salad with 1½ Tbsp low-cal	70	
Small whole-grain roll	80	
Water	0	330 Cal
SNACK		
Fresh fruit in season (peach, plum, etc)	70	
Coffee or tea	10	80 Cal
DINNER		
Meat Loaf (Recipe 4 - page 49)	290	
One-half acorn squash (baked with ½ tsp maple	60	
Spinach (½ cup steamed & drizzled with 1 tsp Evoo)	85	
Romaine lettuce, tomato slices, & 1 Tbsp low-cal	45	
Water	0	495 Cal
SNACK		
Coffee or tea	10	10 Cal
* See Notes - page 13 re using blueberries for raisins		1200 Cal

Day 5 Daily Menu

BREAKFAST	Calories	Totals
Cantaloupe (½ medium)	50	
Fried egg	80	
Toasted raisin bread (1 slice)	75	
Coffee	10	215 Cal
SNACK		
Coffee or tea	10	10 Cal
LUNCH		
Subway 6" (Roast Beef, Cheese + veggies)*	245	
Large tossed salad with 1½ Tbsp low-cal	70	
Hot or iced tea	10	325 Cal
* On 6" half wheat roll.		
SNACK		
Yogurt (6 oz nonfat, any flavor)*	90	
Coffee or tea	10	100 Cal
DINNER		
Frozen fish dinner (Recipe 5 - page 50)	340	
Large tossed salad with 1½ Tbsp low-cal	70	
Whole-grain bread (1 slice)	70	
Fresh fruit in season (apple, peach, etc)	70	
Water	0	550 Cal
SNACK		
Coffee or tea	10	10 Cal
* For example, Dannon Lite & Fit. Buy 32 oz use 6 oz.		1210 Cal

Day 6 Daily Menu

BREAKFAST	Calories	Totals
Tomato juice (½ cup)	20	
Shredded Wheat (1 cup) + ½ cup milk + ½ banana	265	
Coffee	10	295 Cal
SNACK		
Coffee or tea	10	10 Cal
LUNCH		
Leftover meat loaf (½ of Recipe 4) with ketchup	155	
Small whole-grain roll	80	
Lettuce	0	
Fresh or frozen berries (½ cup)	50	
Water	0	285 Cal
SNACK		
Coffee or tea	10	10 Cal
DINNER		
Pizza (Recipe 6 - page 51)	350	
Large tossed salad with 1½ Tbsp low-cal	85	
Fresh fruit in season (apple, plum, etc)	70	
Water	0	550 Cal
SNACK		
Yogurt (4 oz, non-fat any flavor)*	60	
Coffee or tea	10	70 Cal
* Such as Dannon Lite & Fit. Buy 32 oz container use 6 oz.		1210 Cal

Day 7 Daily Menu

BREAKFAST	Calories	Totals
Cantaloupe (½ medium)	50	
Oatmeal ½ cup dry + ½ cup skim milk + 15 raisins	220	
Coffee	10	280 Cal
SNACK		
Coffee or tea	10	10 Cal
LUNCH		
Soup (Appendix B - page 76)	90	
Grilled cheese sandwich (2 slices 2% cheese)	240	
Lettuce and sliced tomato	20	
Pickle spear	0	
Hot or iced tea	10	360 Cal
SNACK		
Coffee or tea	10	10 Cal
DINNER		
Eat Out – Chicken dinner (Recipe 7 - page 52)		
Max allowable calories	530	
Water	0	530 Cal
SNACK		
Coffee or tea	10	10 Cal
		1200 Cal

Day 8 Daily Menu

BREAKFAST	Calories	Totals
Cantaloupe (½ medium)	50	
Wheaties (¾ cup) + ½ cup skim milk + ½ banana	190	
Coffee	10	250 Cal
SNACK		
Fresh fruit in season (peach, plum, etc)	70	
Coffee or tea	10	80 Cal
LUNCH		
Soup (Appendix B - page 76)	130	
Turkey (1 oz) on 1 slice rye bread (½ sandwich)	120	
Lettuce & tomato slices	20	
Hot or iced tea	10	280 Cal
SNACK		
Coffee or tea	10	10 Cal
DINNER		
Baked salmon with salsa (Recipe 8 - page 53)	215	
Baked summer squash and zucchini	40	
Medium tomato - sliced	20	
Brown rice (½ cup – after cooking)	100	
Large tossed salad with 1½ Tbsp low-cal	70	
Water with lemon wedge	10	455 Cal
SNACK		
Graham crackers (3 squares)	90	
Skim milk (4 oz)	45	135 Cal
		1210 Cal

Day 9 Daily Menu

BREAKFAST	Calories	Totals
Orange juice (½ cup)	50	
Soft-boiled egg	80	
Whole grain toast (1 slice)	70	
Coffee	10	210 Cal
SNACK		
Yogurt (6 oz nonfat, any flavor)	90	
Coffee or tea	10	100 Cal
LUNCH		
Salad (3 oz canned tuna, 1 tsp Evoo, onions, celery)	175	
Lettuce & tomato wedges + rye bread (1 slice)	90	
Coffee or tea	10	275 Cal
SNACK		
Handful unsalted mixed nuts	100	
Coffee or tea	10	110 Cal
DINNER		
Veggie burger – (1 patty) (Recipe 9 - page 54)	100	
Low-fat cheddar cheese (1 thin slice)	50	
Seeded hamburger roll	140	
Beets (3 small, boiled, skinned & sliced)	45	
Fresh fruit in season (apple, peach, etc)	70	
Water	0	405 Cal
SNACK		
100-Calorie Pack Cookies	100	
Coffee or tea	10	110 Cal
		1210 Cal

Day 10 Daily Menu

BREAKFAST	Calories	Totals
Orange juice (½ cup)	50	
Wild blueberry pancakes (Recipe 10 - page 55)	190	
Light syrup (1½ Tbsp)	45	
Coffee	10	295 Cal
SNACK		
Coffee or tea	10	10 Cal
LUNCH		
Peanut butter 2 Tbsp on 2 slices whole-grain bread	340	
Skim milk (6 oz)	65	
Fresh fruit in season (apple, plum, etc)	70	475 Cal
SNACK		
Coffee or tea	10	10 Cal
DINNER		
Broiled pork chop about 4 oz meat - trimmed of fat	260	
Green peas (½ cup)	55	
Tomato & cucumber salad 1½ Tbsp low-cal dressing	70	
Water with lemon wedge	10	395 Cal
SNACK		
Coffee or tea	10	10 Cal
		1195 Cal

Day 11 Daily Menu

BREAKFAST	Calories	Totals
Fresh sliced orange	75	
Cheerios (1 cup) + ½ cup skim milk + 15 raisins	190	
Coffee	10	275 Cal
SNACK		
Coffee or tea	10	10 Cal
LUNCH		
Ham & Cheddar*	270	
Fresh fruit in season (apple, plum, etc)	70	
Diet soda or water	0	340 Cal
* Hot Pockets (wrap) or an equivalent food.		
SNACK		
Handful unsalted mixed nuts	100	
Coffee or tea	10	110 Cal
DINNER		
Grilled chicken sausage (2 links 2½ oz per link)	180	
Artichoke-bean salad (Recipe 11 - page 56)	190	
Green beans (¼ lb – steamed)	25	
Whole-grain bread (1 slice)	70	
Water	0	465 Cal
SNACK		
Coffee or tea	10	10 Cal
		1210 Cal

Day 12   Daily Menu

BREAKFAST	Calories	Totals
Orange juice (½ cup)	50	
Scrambled egg	80	
Whole-grain toast (1 slice)	70	
Coffee	10	210 Cal
SNACK		
Yogurt (6 oz nonfat, any flavor)	90	
Coffee or tea	10	100 Cal
LUNCH		
Soup (Appendix B - page 76)	150	
Tomato slices w ¼ cup chopped basil + 1 tsp Evoo	60	
Whole-grain bread (1 slice)	70	
Hot or iced tea	10	290 Cal
SNACK		
Coffee or tea	10	10 Cal
DINNER		
Eat Out – Fish dinner (Recipe 12 - page 57)		
Max allowable calories	595	595 Cal
SNACK		
Coffee or tea	10	10 Cal
		1215 Cal

Day 13 Daily Menu

BREAKFAST	Calories	Totals
Orange juice (½ cup)	50	
Shredded Wheat (1 cup) + ½ cup + ½ banana	260	
Coffee	10	320 Cal
SNACK		
Handful unsalted mixed nuts	100	
Coffee or tea	10	110 Cal
LUNCH		
Turkey frank (2 oz) with mustard & relish	150	
Hot-dog bun	130	
Hot or iced tea	10	290 Cal
SNACK		
Coffee or tea	10	10 Cal
DINNER		
Pasta w Marinara sauce (Recipe 13 - page 58)	225	
Large tossed salad w 1½ Tbsp low-cal dressing	70	
Fresh fruit in season (peach, plum, etc)	70	
Italian or French bread (1 slice)	80	
Water with lemon wedge	10	455 Cal
SNACK		
Coffee or tea	10	10 Cal
		1195 Cal

Day 14 Daily Menu

BREAKFAST	Calories	Totals
Cantaloupe (½ medium)	50	
Low-Cal Smoothie (Recipe 14 - page 59)	220	
Coffee	10	280 Cal
SNACK		
Fresh fruit in season (apple, peach, etc)	70	
Coffee or tea	10	80 Cal
LUNCH		
Grilled Swiss cheese sandwich (2 oz low-fat cheese)	320	
Pickle spear	0	
Hot or iced tea	10	330 Cal
SNACK		
Coffee or tea	10	10 Cal
DINNER		
Frozen chicken dinner (Day 28 Recipe - page 73)	300	
Large tossed salad w 1½ Tbsp low-cal dressing	70	
Water with lemon wedge	10	380 Cal
SNACK		
Popcorn Mini Bag*	110	
Coffee or tea	10	120 Cal
* Such as Orville Redenbacher's Smart Pop		1200 Cal

Day 15 Daily Menu

BREAKFAST	Calories	Totals
Fresh or frozen strawberries (1 cup)	50	
French toasted English Muffin Recipe 3 - page 79	270	
Light syrup (1 Tbsp)	30	
Coffee	10	360 Cal
SNACK		
Yogurt (6 oz nonfat, any flavor)	90	
Coffee or tea	10	100 Cal
LUNCH		
Salad (3 oz canned tuna, 1 tsp Evoo, onions, celery)	175	
Rye bread (1 slice)	70	
Coffee or tea	10	255 Cal
SNACK		
Coffee or tea	10	10 Cal
DINNER		
London broil (Recipe 15 - page 60)	320	
Brown rice (½ cup – after cooking)	100	
Steamed broccoli (1 cup – after cooking)	50	
Water	0	470 Cal
SNACK		
Coffee or tea	10	10 Cal
		1205 Cal

Day 16 Daily Menu

BREAKFAST	Calories	Totals
Orange juice (½ cup)	50	
Kashi GoLean (1 cup) + ½ cup milk + ½ banana	235	
Coffee	10	295 Cal
SNACK		
Fresh fruit in season (apple, plum, etc)	70	
Coffee or tea	10	80 Cal
LUNCH		
Soup (Appendix B - page 76)	100	
Small whole-grain roll	80	
Lettuce and sliced tomato (with 1 Tbsp light mayo)	45	
Hot or iced tea	10	235 Cal
SNACK		
Coffee or tea	10	10 Cal
DINNER		
Baked red snapper (Recipe 16 - page 61)	215	
Wild rice mix (Recipe 16)	160	
Green beans & tomato	75	
Water	0	450 Cal
SNACK		
Popcorn Mini Bag	110	
Coffee or tea	10	120 Cal
		1190 Cal

<u>Day 17 Daily Menu</u>

BREAKFAST	Calories	Totals
Cantaloupe (½ medium)	50	
Fried egg	80	
Toasted raisin bread (1 slice)	75	
Coffee	10	215 Cal
SNACK		
Yogurt (6 oz nonfat, any flavor)	90	
Coffee or tea	10	100 Cal
LUNCH		
Hot Pockets Ham & Cheddar Wrap	270	
Fresh fruit in season (peach, plum, etc)	70	
Cucumber slices and carrots and celery sticks	15	
Hot or iced tea	10	365 Cal
SNACK		
Handful unsalted mixed nuts	100	
Coffee or tea	10	110 Cal
DINNER		
Cajun chicken salad (Recipe 17 - page 62)	330	
Whole-grain bread (1 slice)	70	
Water	0	400 Cal
SNACK		
Coffee or tea	10	10 Cal
		1200 Cal

Day 18 Daily Menu

BREAKFAST	Calories	Totals
Grapefruit (½)	75	
Cheerios (1 cup) + ½ cup skim milk + 15 raisins	190	
Coffee	10	275 Cal
SNACK		
Coffee or tea	10	10 Cal
LUNCH		
Subway 6" (Roast Beef, Cheese + veggies)*	245	
Water (or diet soda)	0	245 Cal
* On 6" half wheat roll.		
SNACK		
Handful unsalted mixed nuts	100	
Coffee or tea	10	110 Cal
DINNER		
Grilled swordfish (**Recipe 18** - page 63)	250	
Grilled potatoes (Recipe 18)	100	
Grilled cherry tomatoes (Recipe 18)	45	
Spinach (½ cup) steamed w garlic & drizzled Evoo	50	
Water with lemon wedge	10	455 Cal
SNACK		
Fiber One Chocolate Fudge Brownie	90	
Coffee or tea	10	100 Cal
		1190 Cal

Day 19 Daily Menu

BREAKFAST	Calories	Totals
Grapefruit (½)	75	
Scrambled egg	80	
Whole-grain toast (1 slice)	70	
Coffee	10	235 Cal
SNACK		
Yogurt (6 oz nonfat, any flavor)	90	
Coffee or tea	10	100 Cal
LUNCH		
Soup (Appendix B - page 197)	90	
Turkey (1 oz) on 1 slice rye bread (½ sandwich)	120	210 Cal
Water	0	
SNACK		
Coffee or tea	10	10 Cal
DINNER		
Eat Out – Chinese food (Recipe 19 - page 64)*		
Max allowable calories	640	640 Cal
SNACK		
Coffee or tea	10	10 Cal
* Bring some home for Day 20 lunch.		1205 Cal

Day 20 Daily Menu

BREAKFAST	Calories	Totals
Tomato juice (½ cup)	20	
Shredded Wheat (1 cup) + ½ cup milk + ½ banana	260	
Coffee	10	290 Cal
SNACK		
Handful unsalted mixed nuts	100	
Coffee or tea	10	110 Cal
LUNCH		
Left over Chinese food from Day 19	260	
Hot or iced tea	10	270 Cal
SNACK		
Coffee or tea	10	10 Cal
DINNER		
Quick Pasta Puttanesca (Recipe 20 - page 65)	345	
Large tossed salad w 1½ Tbsp low-cal dressing	70	
Italian or French bread (1 slice)	80	
Water with lemon wedge	10	505 Cal
SNACK		
Coffee or tea	10	10 Cal
		1195 Cal

Day 21 Daily Menu

BREAKFAST	Calories	Totals
Cantaloupe (½ medium)	50	
Oatmeal ½ cup dry + ½ cup milk + about 15 raisins	220	
Coffee	10	280 Cal
SNACK		
Coffee or tea	10	10 Cal
LUNCH		
Turkey breast (2 oz) on 2 slices bread	245	
Lettuce, tomato and Tbsp light mayo	35	
Pickle spear	0	
Fresh fruit in season (peach, plum, etc)	70	
Water	0	350 Cal
SNACK		
Yogurt (6 oz nonfat, any flavor)	90	
Coffee or tea	10	100 Cal
DINNER		
Frozen meat dinner (Recipe 21 - page 66)	300	
Large tossed salad w 1½ Tbsp low-cal dressing	70	
Whole-grain bread (1 slice)	70	
Water with lemon wedge	10	450 Cal
SNACK		
Coffee or tea	10	10 Cal
		1200 Cal

Day 22 Daily Menu

BREAKFAST	Calories	Totals
Fresh or frozen strawberries (1 cup)	25	
French toasted English Muffin (Recipe 3 - page 109)	270	
Light syrup (1 Tbsp)	30	
Coffee	10	335 Cal
SNACK		
Coffee or tea	10	10 Cal
LUNCH		
Chorizo Egg & Cheese*	260	
Hot or iced tea	10	270 Cal
* Hot Pockets wrap or an equivalent food.		
SNACK		
Yogurt (6 oz nonfat, any flavor)	90	
Coffee or tea	10	100 Cal
DINNER		
Shrimp & spinach salad (Recipe 22 - page 67)	310	
Whole-grain bread (1 slice)	70	
Fresh fruit in season (apple, peach, etc)	70	
Water with lemon wedge	10	460 Cal
SNACK		
Coffee or tea	10	10 Cal
		1185 Cal

Day 23 Daily Menu

BREAKFAST	Calories	Totals
Cantaloupe (½ medium)	50	
Wheaties (¾ cup) + ½ cup skim milk + ½ banana	190	
Coffee	10	250 Cal
SNACK		
Handful unsalted mixed nuts	100	
Coffee or tea	10	110 Cal
LUNCH		
Ham (2 oz) w mustard on 2 slices rye bread	300	
Pickle spear	0	
Hot or iced tea	10	315 Cal
SNACK		
Coffee or tea	10	10 Cal
DINNER		
Beans & Greens Salad (Recipe 23 - page 68)	260	
Whole-grain bread (1 slice)	70	
Baked potato (medium)	100	
Fresh fruit in season (apple, plum, etc)	70	
Water	0	500 Cal
SNACK		
Coffee or tea	10	10 Cal
		1195 Cal

Day 24 Daily Menu

BREAKFAST	Calories	Totals
Fresh orange sliced	75	
Soft-boiled egg	80	
Whole grain toast (1 slice)	70	
Coffee	10	235 Cal
SNACK		
Yogurt (6 oz nonfat, any flavor)	90	
Coffee or tea	10	100 Cal
LUNCH		
Salad 3 oz canned salmon, 1 tsp Evoo, onions celery	200	
Lettuce & tomato wedges	20	
Rye bread (1 slice)	70	
Coffee or tea	10	300 Cal
SNACK		
Fresh fruit in season (peach, plum, etc)	70	
Coffee or tea	10	80 Cal
DINNER		
Chicken breast (5 oz - skinless, broiled)	250	
Four bean salad (½ cup) (Recipe 24 - page 69)	135	
Large tossed salad with 1½ Tbsp low-cal	70	
Water with lemon wedge	10	465 Cal
SNACK		
Coffee or tea	10	10 Cal
		1190 Cal

<h1 align="center"><u>Day 25 Daily Menu</u></h1>

BREAKFAST	Calories	Totals
Grapefruit (½)	75	
Cheerios (1 cup) + ½ cup skim milk + 15 raisins	190	
Coffee	10	275 Cal
SNACK		
Coffee or tea	10	10 Cal
LUNCH		
Cottage cheese (1 cup low fat)	180	
Large tossed salad w 1½ Tbsp low-cal dressing	70	
Small whole-grain roll	80	
Hot or iced tea	10	340 Cal
SNACK		
Coffee or tea	10	10 Cal
DINNER		
Hanger steak (Recipe 25 - page 70)	320	
Roasted potatoes (Recipe 25)	120	
Cherry tomatoes (Recipe 25)	20	
Steamed spinach (½ cup)	25	
Whole-grain bread (1 slice)	70	
Water	0	555 Cal
SNACK		
Coffee or tea	10	10 Cal
		1200 Cal

Day 26 Daily Menu

BREAKFAST	Calories	Totals
Cantaloupe (½ medium)	50	
Fried eggs (2 eggs)	160	
Toasted whole-grain bread (1 slice)	70	
Coffee	10	290 Cal
SNACK		
Yogurt (6 oz nonfat, any flavor)	90	
Coffee or tea	10	100 Cal
LUNCH		
Soup (Appendix B - page 76)	160	
Hard whole-grain roll (medium)	80	
Lettuce & tomato slices	20	
Hot or iced tea	10	270 Cal
SNACK		
Fresh fruit in season (apple, peach, etc)	70	
Coffee or tea	10	80 Cal
DINNER		
Grilled scallops (Recipe 26 - page 71)	210	
Grilled polenta (Recipe 26)	125	
Mushroom-steamed green beans-red onion	45	
Grilled asparagus (as shown in Recipe 26)	10	
Large tossed salad w 1½ Tbsp low-cal dressing	70	
Water	0	460 Cal
SNACK		
Coffee or tea	10	10 Cal
		1210 Cal

Day 27 Daily Menu

BREAKFAST	Calories	Totals
Orange juice (½ cup)	50	
Oatmeal ½ cup dry + ½ cup skim milk + 15 raisins	220	
Coffee	10	280 Cal
SNACK		
Coffee or tea	10	10 Cal
LUNCH		
Left over Bean Salad from Day 23 (1 serving)	260	
Small whole-grain roll	80	
Lettuce & tomato slices	20	
Hot or iced tea	10	370 Cal
SNACK		
Fresh fruit in season (apple, plum, etc)	70	
Coffee or tea	10	80 Cal
DINNER		
Fettuccine (Recipe 27 - page 72)	290	
Large tossed salad w 1½ Tbsp low-cal dressing	70	
Italian or French bread (1 slice)	80	
Water with lemon wedge	10	450 Cal
SNACK		
Coffee or tea	10	10 Cal
		1200 Cal

Day 28 Daily Menu

BREAKFAST	Calories	Totals
Cantaloupe (½ medium)	50	
Smoothie (Recipe 14 - page 90)	220	
Coffee	10	280 Cal
SNACK		
Fresh fruit in season (peach, plum, etc)	70	
Coffee or tea	10	80 Cal
LUNCH		
Roast beef (2 oz) sandwich on whole-grain bread	295	
Lettuce	0	
Pickle spear	0	
Hot or iced tea	10	305 Cal
SNACK		
Coffee or tea	10	10 Cal
DINNER		
Frozen chicken dinner (Recipe 28 - page 73)	300	
Large tossed salad w 1½ Tbsp low-cal dressing	70	
Whole-grain bread (1 slice)	70	
Water	0	
Fiber One Chocolate Fudge Brownie	90	530 Cal
SNACK		
Coffee or tea	10	10 Cal
		1215 Cal

Day 29 Daily Menu

BREAKFAST	Calories	Totals
Orange juice (½ cup)	50	
Wild blueberry pancakes (Recipe 10 - page 24)	190	
Light syrup (1½ Tbsp)	45	
Coffee	10	295 Cal
SNACK		
Yogurt (6 oz nonfat, any flavor)	90	
Coffee or tea	10	100 Cal
LUNCH		
Salad (3 oz canned tuna, 1 tsp Evoo, onions, celery)	175	
Lettuce & tomato wedges	20	
Rye bread (1 slice)	70	
Fresh fruit in season (apple, pear, etc)	70	
Coffee or tea	10	345 Cal
SNACK		
Coffee or tea	10	10 Cal
DINNER		
Barbequed shrimp (Recipe 29 - page 74)	160	
Corn on the cob (medium)	90	
Steamed broccoli (1 cup – after cooking)	50	
Water	0	300 Cal
SNACK		
Kashi TLC Chewy Granola Bar	140	
Coffee or tea	10	150 Cal
		1200 Cal

Day 30 Daily Menu

BREAKFAST	Calories	Totals
Fresh orange sliced	75	
Kashi GoLean (1 cup) + ½ cup milk + ½ banana	235	
Coffee	10	320 Cal
SNACK		
Fresh fruit in season (apple, plum, etc)	70	
Coffee or tea	10	80 Cal
LUNCH		
Soup (Appendix B - page 76)	130	
Small whole-grain roll	80	
Raw zucchini slices, celery and carrot sticks	20	
Water	0	230 Cal
SNACK		
Coffee or tea	10	10 Cal
DINNER		
Cheeseburger (Recipe 30 - page 75)	370	
Lettuce and sliced tomato	20	
Whole-grain hard roll	140	
Steamed green beans	25	
Pickle spear	0	
Water	0	555 Cal
SNACK		
Coffee or tea	10	10 Cal
		1205 Cal

Recipes and Diet Tips

Day 1- Recipe

<u>Chicken with Peppers & Onions</u>

   4 boneless and skinless chicken breasts (about 5 oz each)
Coat the chicken breasts in a bottled barbeque sauce. Prepare medium-hot fire on well-oiled grill. Place breasts on grill, turning them every 4 minutes, for 10 to 12 minutes, or until done. (To check if breasts are done, the meat should be moist and white with no sign of pink when you cut into the breast.) Salt and pepper to taste.
   2 medium red peppers, sliced
   1 medium onion, sliced
Place peppers and onions in pan with 2 tablespoons fat-free chicken stock. Sauté until stock is reduced. Spray pan lightly with non-stick cooking oil and cook another 2 minutes. Salt and pepper to taste.
<u>Serves 4</u>. About 250 Calories per serving (for chicken only).

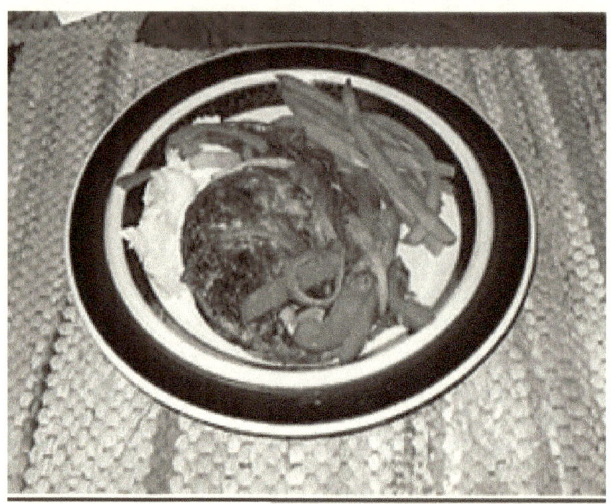

<u>Diet Tip of the Day:</u> Weight Loss – take it one step, one meal, one workout, one day at a time. Just think of where you'll be in 90 days!

Day 2 - Recipe

<u>Baked Herb-Crusted Cod</u>

4 cod fish fillets (4 to 5 ounces each)
2 tablespoons flour
2 tablespoons cornmeal
2 tablespoons minced fresh herbs
2 teaspoons lemon juice

Sprinkle cod with lemon juice. Mix flour, cornmeal and herbs and dust the cod with the cornmeal-herb mixture. Bake in oven at 375 ºF for 10 minutes. Add salt and black pepper to taste.

<u>Serves 4</u>. One serving is about 230 Calories (for cod only).

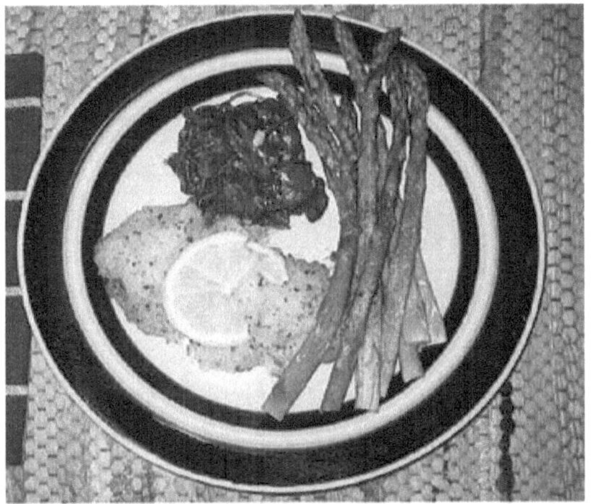

<u>Diet Tip of the Day:</u>. A **reducing diet is best supervised by a physician**. This is especially true when a great deal of weight needs to be lost, or if you have an ailment or a history of medical problems.

Day 3 - Recipe

French-Toasted English Muffin

   6 whole wheat light English muffins, sliced in half
   4 eggs
   2 cups skim milk
   2 teaspoons vanilla
   A dash of cinnamon

In a medium bowl, beat together eggs and skim milk. Add vanilla and cinnamon. Slice English muffins into halves and saturate slices in egg mixture. In a non-stick skillet coated with cooking spray, cook muffins until both sides are golden brown. Dust lightly with confectionary sugar. Serve hot or keep in an oven or warmer at 200 ºF until ready to plate. **Serves 4**. Three English muffin slices per serving. Serving is 270 Calories.

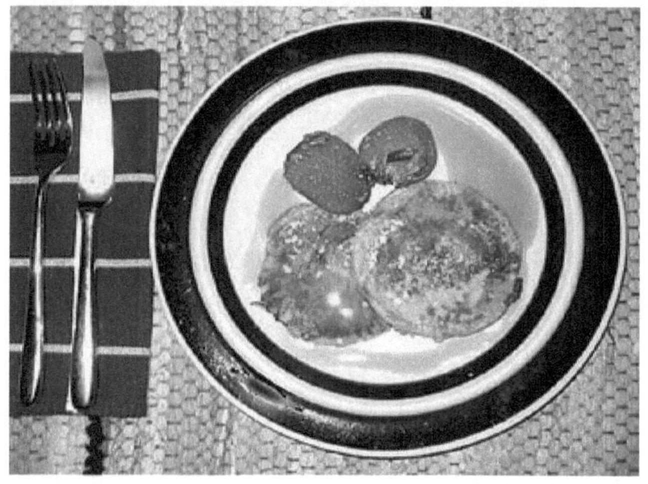

Diet Tip of the Day: **"Eat Slowly"** This is especially vital when you are trying to lose weight. If you are someone who eats fast, who finishes before everyone else at the table, you are not giving yourself a chance to feel full. While everyone else is still eating, you either sit there and pick, or you have seconds, taking in extra calories you could avoid if you would just slow down.

Day 4 - Recipe

Carrie's Low-Cal Meat Loaf

½ pound ground white meat turkey
½ pound ground beef (about 90% lean)
1 large egg
½ cup skim milk
¼ cup bread crumbs
¼ cup ketchup
¼ cup chopped carrots
¼ cup chopped onion
In a medium bowl, combine all ingredients. Add salt and pepper to taste. Mix until blended and form into a loaf. Place loaf into oven preheated to 350 °F. Bake until an instant-read thermometer inserted in the center of the loaf reads 160 °F. This should take about one hour.

Shown below is meat loaf, acorn squash (baked with 1 teaspoon of maple syrup). Also shown is steamed spinach drizzled with extra-virgin olive oil.
Serves 5. About 290 Calories per serving (for meat loaf only). Note: reserve half a serving of the meat loaf which is to be eaten for lunch on Day 6.

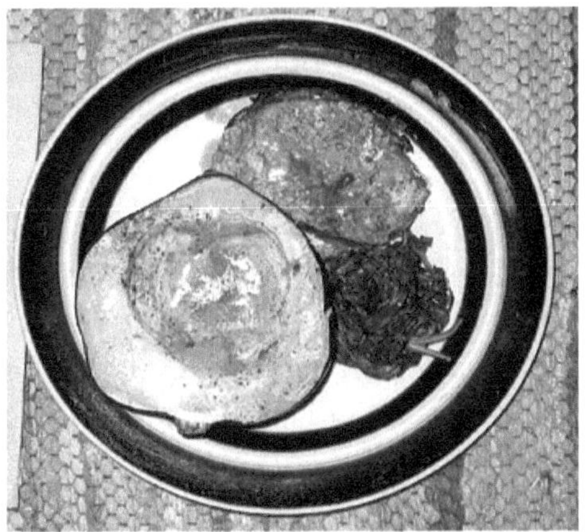

Diet Tip of the Day: **Take a daily multi-vitamin/mineral supplement.** This is very important when you're on a diet – as a kind of insurance policy.

Day 5 - Recipe

Frozen-Fish Dinner

No recipe today. No cooking today. It's your day off! Some reasonably good frozen fish dinners are:

Shrimp Alfredo	**Lean Cuisine**	~~230~~ 240
Tuna Noodle Casserole	**Smart Ones**	~~250~~ 270
Shrimp & Angel Hair Pasta	**Lean Cuisine**	~~280~~ 290
Parmesan Crusted Fish	**Lean Cuisine**	~~290~~ 300
Tortilla Crusted Fish	**Lean Cuisine**	~~300~~ 310

That's it. At this writing, there are just not that many frozen fish dinners for sale at supermarkets, although new entrees are being introduced continually. If you choose any of the above entrees, you will not use all of the **340 Calories allocated for this meal**. In this case, use the excess calories anyway you wish. Splurge on extra dessert or save the calories for another day!

See **Appendix B** on page 198 for our comprehensive list of frozen entrees. Please read the important **Frozen-Food Safety Warning** in **Appendix C** on page 203.

<u>Diet Tip of the Day:</u> **Buy a pedometer** and start walking. For the average person 2100 steps amounts to walking about one mile. A Harvard study has shown that 8000 to 10,000 step per day promote weight loss. And you're not obliged to walk continuously until you accrue all 10,000 steps. Rather, all steps throughout the day to wherever and whenever count toward your daily total. Because 10,000 steps a day may not be achievable by some people, particularly those who are elderly, sedentary, or who have chronic diseases, rather than insisting on a blanket 10,000 steps per day, your initial stepping goal should your baseline steps plus an increment of an additional 2500 steps . (Your baseline being the number of steps you take in an average day.)

<h1 style="text-align:center">Day 6 - Recipe</h1>

<u>Grandma's Pizza</u>

The following is a pizza recipe used by Gail Johnson's Italian grandmother. She was from a small mountain village located between Rome and Naples.

Pizza dough: To save time use prepared dough, preferably whole wheat. To start, flour a large cutting board. Divide one pound of prepared pizza dough into four parts. Roll out each dough ball as thin as possible.

Tomato sauce: Sauté ½ small onion, chopped fine, in 1 teaspoon olive oil. Add two finely chopped garlic cloves, 1½ cups chopped plum tomatoes and ½ teaspoon chopped fresh oregano. Stir and cook about 5 minutes on a low flame.

Pizza preparation & cooking: On each pizza, spread evenly ¼ cup of the tomato sauce. Add ½ ounce of shredded part-skim mozzarella cheese, 1 teaspoon Parmesan cheese, 3 slices of a Portobello mushroom, some torn fresh basil, and drizzle with extra-virgin olive oil. Put pizzas on a pan and place in 475 °F oven for about 15 to 20 minutes, or until crust is crisp and cheese is just melting. (Freeze left over sauce for use on Day 13.)

<u>Serves 4</u>. Each pizza contains approximately 350 Calories.

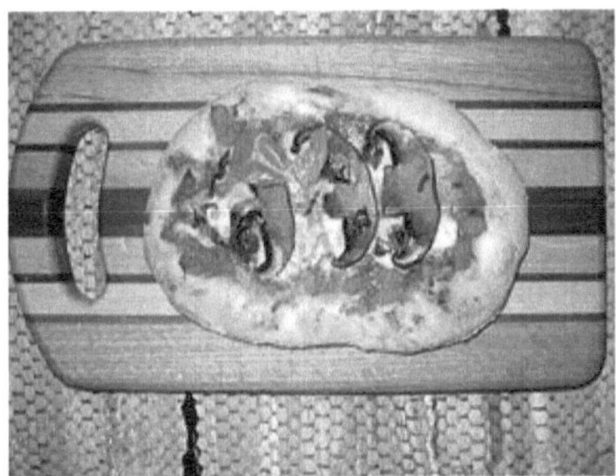

<u>Diet Tip of the Day:</u> For **life-long weight control** take a vigorous 30 to 60 minute walk everyday! That's right – everyday. Make exercise a nonflexible top priority part of your life. When it comes to exercise the key words are consistent, persistent, unyielding, dogged. Get the point?

51

Day 7 - Recipe

<u>Chicken Dinner - Out</u>

No recipe today. No cooking today. Have a chicken dinner at your favorite restaurant, but make sure you choose a restaurant where you have a fighting chance to achieve your calorie goal. For your chicken dinner out, your maximum allowable calories (includes appetizer, soup, main course and dessert) are as follows:

- For the **1200 Calorie Diet**: 530 Calories
- For the **1500 Calorie Diet**: 630 Calories
- For the **1800 Calorie Diet**: 630 Calories

Tips for Eating Chicken Out: First, order simple and order skinless white meat only, such as broiled chicken breast with steamed vegetables and brown rice. Tell the waiter you want no sauce, no gravy, nothing added. Then, knowing your calorie objective, and that chicken is about 50 Calories per ounce, most steamed vegetable servings average approximately 50 Calories per cup, and rice is about 100 Calories per ½ cup, decide how much to eat – and take the remainder home. If fresh fruit is not an option, pass on dessert and have the evening snack specified for that day in this diet.

In a restaurant, most nutritionists recommend you eat the low-calorie items on your plate first. Start with the salad, soup and veggies. By the time you get to the chicken and starches you will hopefully be full enough to be content with smaller portions of the higher-calorie choices. (Incidentally, feel free to substitute skinless white meat turkey for chicken.)

Finally, some dieticians advise their dieting clients not to eat out. That's right. They believe eating at home is safer. But our thought is you have to eat out eventually so why not learn how while your resolve is high?

<u>Diet Tip of the Day:</u> When you're on a diet, eating in a restaurant can be a challenge, because most restaurant portions are huge, and can easily total more than 1000 Calories. So, in a restaurant decide how much to eat – and take the remainder home. A good general rule of thumb is to **eat half and bring the rest home**.

Day 8 - Recipe

<u>Baked Salmon with Salsa</u>

This is a simple, straight-forward recipe. The advantage of a simple recipe is there are no hidden calories.

4   5 oz salmon fillets

6   tablespoons bottled tomato-pepper salsa

Brown salmon fillets in non-stick pan and then place them in a baking dish. Cook fillets in an oven preheated to 350 °F for about 10 minutes. Plate the salmon. Stir bottled tomato-pepper salsa and spoon it over the salmon.

<u>Serves 4</u>. One salmon fillet is about 215 Calories.

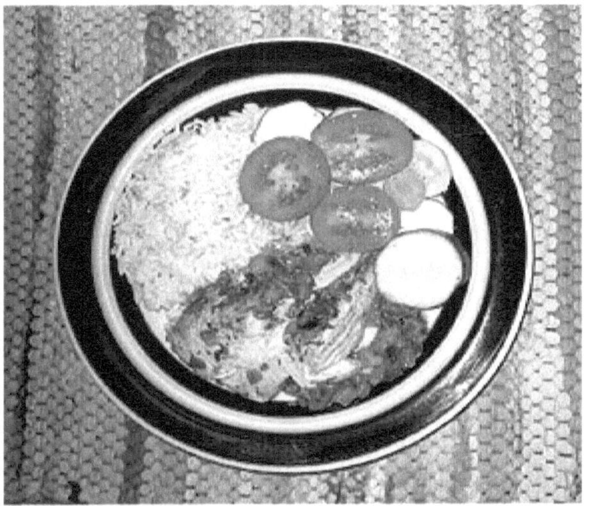

<u>Diet Tip of the Day:</u> Hunger is your body's way of telling you that you need calories. But **when you're done eating, you should feel better – satisfied but not stuffed**.

Day 9 - Recipe

<u>Veggie Burger</u>

Vegetable-based burgers can be purchased at your local supermarket. Patties of a veggie burger are made from either vegetables, soy, nuts, mushrooms, textured vegetable protein, dairy, or a combination of these foods.

In the U.S., two popular veggie burgers are the Boca Burger and Gardenburger. The Boca Burger is made chiefly from soy protein and wheat gluten. (Boca Burger patties are 2.5 oz each and range from 60 to 90 Calories.) The original Gardenburger is made from mushrooms, onions, brown rice, rolled oats, cheese, and spices. (Gardenburger patties are 2.5 oz each and about 100 Calories.)

To prepare, follow package directions. The version shown below has an added slice of low-fat cheddar cheese. The lettuce, tomato and ketchup shown actually add very few extra calories.

The veggie burger patty plus low-fat cheese amounts to approximately 150 Calories. Add a seeded roll and the total rises to 290 Calories.

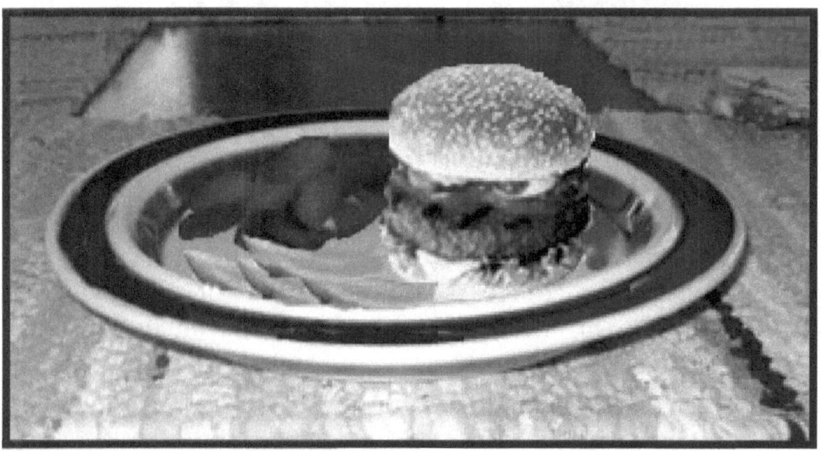

<u>Diet Tip of the Day:</u> **Drink lots of water** – about 8 glasses per day when you're trying to lose weight. Add a slice of lemon to make it more interesting. Often, when you think you're hungry, you are just thirsty. So, next time you crave a snack, drink some water first and see if that does it for you.

Day 10 - Recipe

Wild Blueberry Pancakes

This recipe makes a relatively low calorie, wholesome batch of delicious wild blueberry-whole wheat-buttermilk pancakes.
1 cup whole-wheat flour
1 cup buttermilk
1 egg
1 tablespoon vegetable oil
1 teaspoon baking powder
½ teaspoon baking soda
Stir ingredients until blended. Add ¾ cup fresh of frozen blueberries and gently stir. Using medium heat, preheat a non-stick skillet coated with cooking spray. Pour slightly less than ¼ cup of batter onto skillet per pancake. Cook slowly until bubbles break on surface of pancake. Turn and cook until other side is lightly browned.

Makes 8 pancakes. Pictured below are wild-blueberry pancakes with two slices of turkey bacon.
Serves 4. Each pancake is about 95 Calories

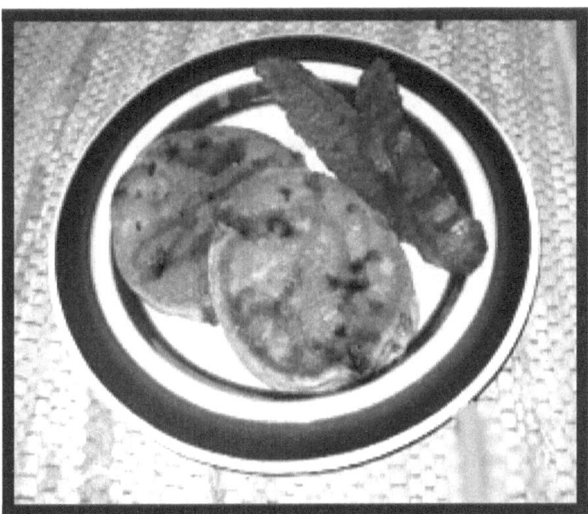

Bacon allowable only on 1500 and 1800 Calorie diets.

Diet Tip of the Day: Most experts associate eating a substantial breakfast with successful weight loss.

Artichoke-Bean Salad

19-ounce can white kidney beans
10 artichoke hearts, quartered
⅓ cup chopped oregano
⅓ cup chopped parsley
3 cloves garlic, chopped
1 lemon, juiced

Combine ingredients in medium-size bowl. Stir in ¼ cup extra-virgin olive oil. Salt and black pepper to taste.
Serves 6. Approximately 190 Calories per serving.

Pictured on the plate below is the artichoke-bean salad as a side dish with two grilled chicken sausage links, tomato salsa and steamed green beans. Incidentally, this artichoke-bean combination over mixed salad greens served with a whole-grain bread makes a delicious, nutritious and reasonable low-calorie main course.

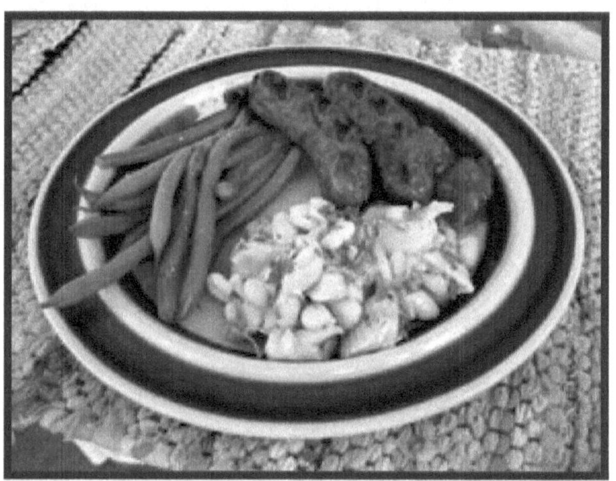

Diet Tip of the Day: Before you go to a **party**, have a small meal, such as a hardboiled egg, an apple, and a thirst quencher (like water, tea, seltzer, or diet soda). This will take the edge off your appetite and make it easier to resist the high-calorie goodies.

Day 12 - Recipe

Fish Dinner - Out

No recipe today. No cooking today. Have a fish dinner at your favorite restaurant, but make sure you choose a restaurant where you have a good chance to achieve your calorie goal. For today, your **goal for dinner is a maximum of 595 Calories**. This includes appetizer, soup, main course and dessert.

Tips for Eating Fish Out: The following is almost an exact repeat of the advice given eating out on previous days. First, order simple, such as broiled fish with steamed vegetables and brown rice. Tell the waiter you want no sauce, no gravy, nothing added. Then, knowing your calorie objective, and that fish is about 50 Calories per ounce, most steamed vegetable servings average approximately 50 Calories per cup, and rice is about 100 Calories per ½ cup, decide how much to eat – and take the remainder home. If fresh fruit is not an option, pass on dessert and have the evening snack specified for that day in the diet.

In a restaurant, some nutritionists recommend you eat the low-calorie items on your plate first. Start with the salad, soup and veggies. By the time you get to the fish and starches you will hopefully be full enough to be content with smaller portions of the higher-calorie choices.

Diet Tip of the Day: Phytonutrients are found in plant foods such as fruits, vegetables, whole grains, dried beans, nuts and seeds. Unlike protein, fat, vitamins and minerals, phytonutrients are not necessary for life, but evidence is growing that phytonutrients have many beneficial qualities.

Day 13 - Recipe

<u>Pasta with Marinara Sauce</u>

Prepare the sauce as you did for the Day 6 pizza (on page 112). But because the pizza sauce is a bit too thick, we add ¼ cup of pasta liquid to thin it. (The spiral pasta profile shown below is called fusilli, a very popular pasta shape because all those ridges hold buckets of tomato sauce.)

    ½ pound <u>whole-wheat</u> pasta
    ¼ teaspoon salt

Prepare the marinara tomato sauce as per Day 6 sauce but dilute it with ¼ cup of today's pasta liquid.

Bring 2 quarts of lightly salted water to a boil. Add pasta and stir occasionally (to keep pasta from sticking to the bottom of the pot). Keep water boiling and cook until pasta are "al dente." (Cooking time is approximately 9 minutes.) Drain pasta, add marinara sauce and serve hot.

<u>Serves 4</u>. One serving is about 225 Calories.

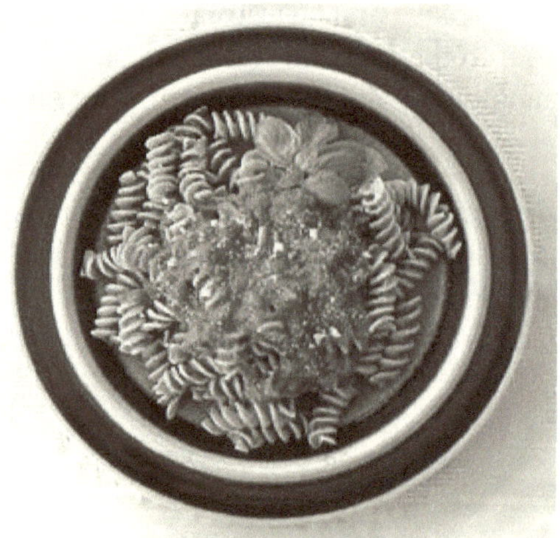

<u>**Diet Tip of the Day:**</u> **Beware of alcoholic beverages**. Beer has about 13 Calories per ounce, wine 25 Calories per ounce and whiskey a whopping 71 Calories per ounce.

Day 14 - Recipe

Low-Cal Smoothie

Smoothies are delicious, nutritious and fun to drink! They're great for a fast but nutritious breakfast, a light energy-boosting lunch, a healthy snack, a late afternoon pick me up, and a delicious dessert. Making your own smoothie is a smart way to save money and get healthy at the same time!

8 ounces plain fat-free yogurt
1 cup orange juice
1 cup strawberries
½ cup blueberries
1 banana
1 teaspoon sugar
1 teaspoon vanilla extract

Place yogurt, strawberries, and blueberries in a blender. Pour in orange juice. Add sugar and vanilla extract to mixture. Blend all ingredients until thick and smooth. Pour smoothie into a glass and enjoy.

Serves 2. About 220 Calories per serving

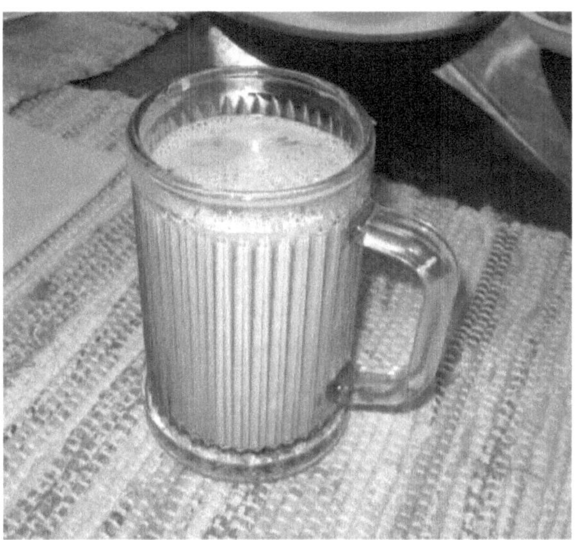

Diet Tip of the Day: Two scientific journals indicate **dark chocolate** - not white chocolate or milk chocolate - is potent antioxidant and is good for you. But don't overdo it, because you have to offset the extra chocolate calories by eating less of other foods.

Day 15 - Recipe

<u>London Broil</u>

    1 lb boneless flank steak about ¾" thick, fat trimmed
    1 clove garlic
    1 teaspoon dry oregano

Rub each side of the flank steak with garlic. Season with oregano, salt and pepper to taste. Prepare a large non-stick skillet over high heat. Steak should sizzle when placed on hot skillet. Sear steak on one side for about 5 minutes; then turn and sear other side for about 4 minutes, or until done to preference. Check the center by making small incision. Carve into ¼-inch slices.

<u>**Serves 4**</u>. About 320 Calories per serving (for meat only).

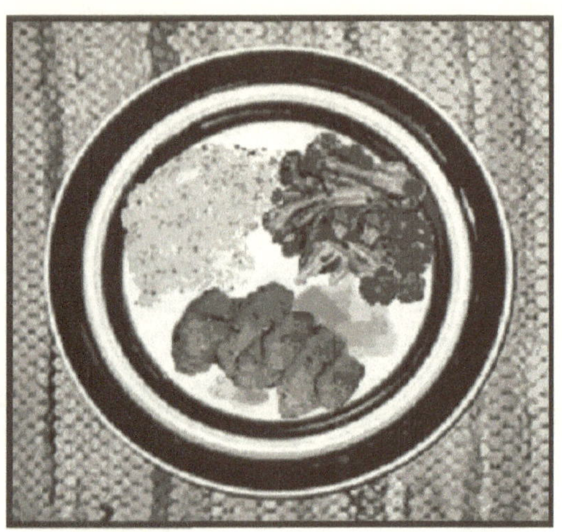

<u>**Diet Tip of the Day:**</u> **Stay Busy.** Most people will do anything to avoid work, housework, yard work, exercise, etc. But any kind of work burns a lot more calories than just sitting! Whatever it is you are avoiding – just go do it!

Day 16 - Recipe

<u>Red Snapper with Special Sauce</u>

    4 4-ounce red snapper fillets (salmon fillets okay)
    ½ cup white wine
    ½ cup non-fat yogurt mixed with ¼ cup mustard
    ½ pound green beans
    ¾ pint cherry tomatoes (about 20), halved
    4 teaspoons olive oil
    ¾ cup wild rice, brown rice and wheat berry mix.

Brown fillets in non-stick pan. Place fillets skin side down in baking dish coated with non-stick spray. Add white wine and cook in oven preheated to 350 ºF for about 15 minutes . Spoon pan juices over fillets. Salt and pepper to taste.

Place green beans in skillet. Add ¼-inch of water and cook over medium heat until water boils off. Add cherry tomatoes and olive oil. Stir well and sauté for a few minutes. (If desired, season with fresh rosemary and oregano.) Salt and pepper to taste.

Prepare rice mix per package directions.

Plate red snapper fillet and spoon over yogurt-mustard sauce. Add green beans and tomato mix and the wild rice mix. Serve hot.
<u>Serves 4.</u> One plate consisting of a snapper fillet (215 Cal) with green beans & tomato mix (75 Cal) and wild rice (160 Cal) totals 450 Calories.

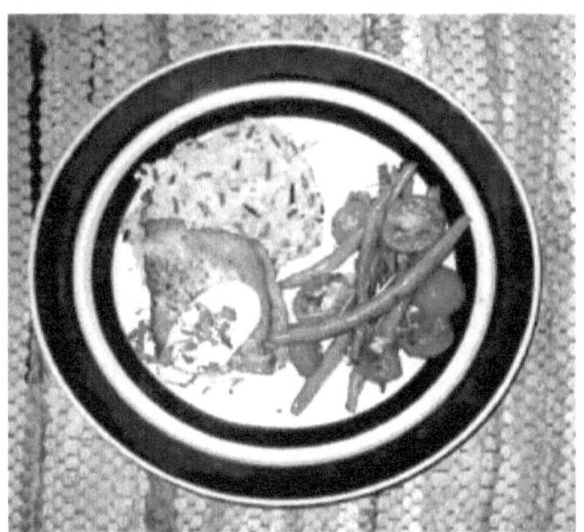

<u>**Diet Tip of the Day:**</u> **Don't have sweets in your house**. This makes them easier to resist. Out of sight, out of mind!

<u>Cajun Chicken Salad</u>

This is a perfect after-work, quick, nutritious and delicious dinner.

- 4 boneless and skinless chicken breasts - about 5 oz each
- 4 teaspoons of bottled Cajun herb-spice mix
- 8 ounces mixed salad greens
- ¾ pint cherry tomatoes (about 20), halved
- 12 pitted black olives
- 2 tablespoons bottled light salad dressing

Brush chicken breasts lightly with olive oil. Roll breasts in Cajun herb-spice mix.

Brown breasts on non-stick oven-proof skillet. After breasts are brown, put skillet in 350 °F oven for approximately 15 minutes, or until done. (When the breasts are done, the meat should be moist and white with no sign of pink.) Cut breasts into ½-inch slices.

Serve hot or keep in an oven or warmer at 200 °F until ready to plate. Place chicken slices over a bed of mixed salad greens. Add tomatoes, olives and two tablespoons of your favorite low-calorie salad dressing. <u>Serves 4</u>. 330 Calories per serving

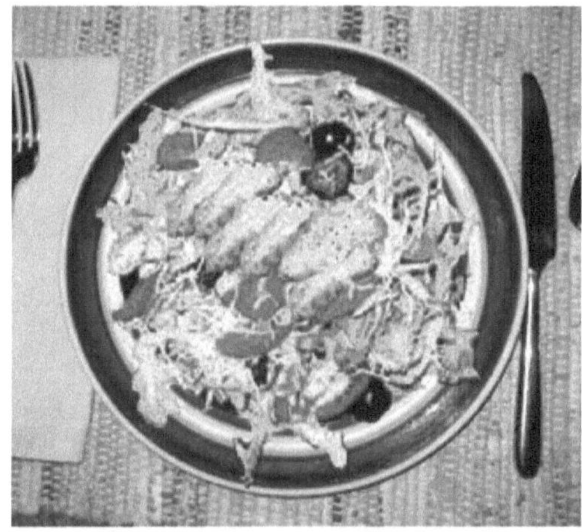

<u>Diet Tip of the Day:</u> Hot or cold cereal topped with fruit, and fat-free milk makes a nutritious, relatively low-calorie meal anytime.

Day 18 - Recipe

Grilled Swordfish

1¼ pounds swordfish
1 bottle citrus-herb marinade
¾ pint cherry tomatoes (about 20), halved
4 medium potatoes
2 cups fresh spinach
1 teaspoon rosemary & juice of ¼ lemon
2 teaspoon extra-virgin olive oil, divided
Steam spinach with garlic and drizzle with about 1 teaspoon extra-virgin olive oil.

Cut potatoes in medium-size pieces and sprinkle with lemon juice, add rosemary, salt and black pepper. Place potatoes on grill for about 10 minutes, turning occasionally.

Toss cherry tomatoes in remaining extra-virgin olive oil. Add fresh oregano, salt and black pepper. Place on heavy-duty aluminum foil, seal and grill for about 3 minutes.

Marinade swordfish in citrus-herb vinaigrette. Grill on hot fire for about 5 minutes on one side and 3 minutes on the other, or until done as desired.
Serves 4. One plate of grilled swordfish (250 Calories) with potatoes (100 Calories), cherry tomatoes (45 Calories) and steamed spinach (50 Calories) totals 445 Calories.

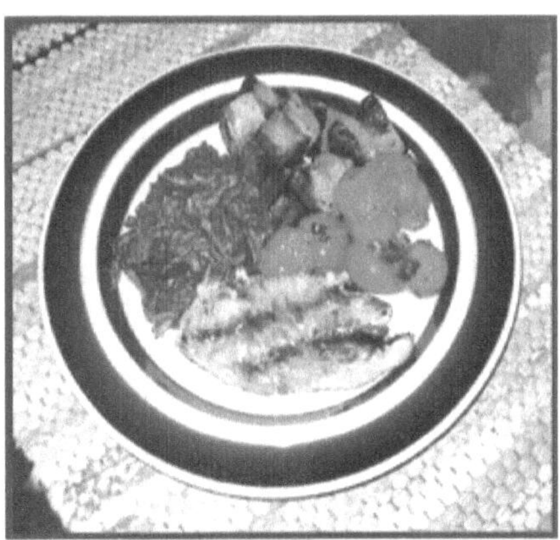

<u>Chinese Dinner - Out</u>

No recipe today. No cooking today. Have a Chinese dinner at your favorite restaurant, but make sure you choose a restaurant where you have a reasonable chance to achieve your calorie goal. For today, **your goal for dinner is a maximum of 640 Calories**. This includes any appetizer, soup, main course and any dessert.

Tips for Eating Chinese: You can consume a lot of calories in a Chinese restaurant – if you order carelessly. For example a typical portion of General Tso's chicken is loaded with about 1000 Calories, then add another 200 Calories for a cup of rice.

First rule, order simple. Look for an entree with lots of vegetables, some fish or chicken and brown rice. Tell the waiter you want your food steamed with any sauce on the side. (This is not only a low-calorie way of eating Chinese food but is also the most nutritious way to eat Chinese food.)

Then, knowing your 640 Calorie objective, and that chicken and fish are about 50 Calories per ounce, most steamed vegetable servings average approximately 50 Calories per cup, and rice is about 200 Calories per cup, decide how much of the meal you can eat – and take the remainder home. (Note that you will be eating half a serving of left over Chinese food for lunch tomorrow.) To stay within your maximum allowable calorie total, you should pass on dessert and have the evening snack specified for that day in the diet.

Incidentally, although Chinese is specified, feel free to substitute Thai food, Vietnamese, Indian, Middle Eastern, or any other favorite ethnic food. Just make sure you don't exceed the maximum allowable 640 calories for this meal.

<u>Diet Tip of the Day:</u> Another dilemma for dieters is **judging portion size**. It makes no sense to worry about whether to apportion 70 or 80 Calories per ounce for a cut of lean meat if you have no idea whether the portion you are planning to eat weighs four or ten ounces. To be successful, you must learn to estimate <u>portion sizes</u> with reasonable accuracy.

Day 20 - Recipe

Quick Pasta alla Puttanesca

This famous pasta dish originated in Naples Italy. Puttanesca means "ladies of the night." Although the exact origin of the name is unclear, one thing is clear: It's delicious! Here is one of many recipe versions.

½ pound spaghetti (whole wheat preferred)

20 black or green pitted olives

14.5-oz can diced tomatoes

4 oz tomato sauce

2 tablespoon extra-virgin olive oil

3 cloves of garlic, chopped

1 tablespoon dried minced onion

½ teaspoon crushed red pepper flakes

1 tablespoon capers drained and rinsed

¼ cup currants

Cook spaghetti according to package directions. Drain and return spaghetti to pot; add a teaspoon extra-virgin olive oil and toss to coat.

Heat remaining olive oil in large skillet over medium-high heat. Add red pepper flakes; cook and stir 1 to 2 minutes or until sizzling. Add onion and garlic; cook and stir 1 minute. Add canned tomatoes with juice, tomato sauce, olives, currants and capers. Cook over medium-high heat, stirring frequently, until sauce is heated through.

Serves 4. About 345 Calories per serving

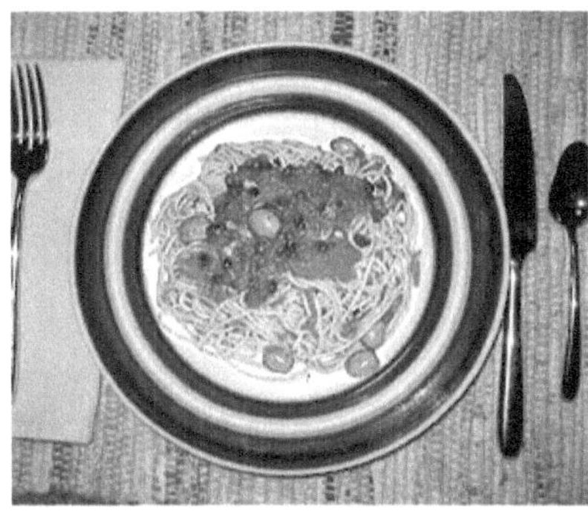

Diet Tip of the Day: Dilute fruit juices, such as apple juice, orange, etc. with water. This cuts the flavor slightly but really reduces calorie content.

Day 21 - Recipe

Frozen-Meat Dinner

No recipe today. No cooking today. Another day off! That's it. At this writing, there are just not that many frozen meat dinners for sale at supermarkets, although new entrees are being introduced continually. Here are some reasonably good frozen-meat dinners:

Steak Portobella	**Lean Cuisine**	160
Asian Style Beef & Broccoli	**Smart Ones**	~~160~~ 170
Beef Merlot	**Healthy Choice**	180
Homestyle Beef Pot Roast	**Smart Ones**	180
Salisbury Steak w Mac & Cheese	**Lean Cuisine**	~~270~~ 290
Pasta with Swedish Meatballs	**Smart Ones**	~~280~~ 290
Classic Meat Loaf	**Healthy Choice**	300

If you choose most of the above entrees, you will fall well short of the **300 Calories allocated for this day**. In this case, use the remaining calories anyway you wish. Indulge on extra dessert or save the calories for another day.

See **Appendix B** on page 198 for our comprehensive list of frozen entrees. Please read the important **Frozen-Food Safety Warning** in **Appendix C** on page 203.

Diet Tip of the Day: **Understanding nutrition** is not only vital for good health but also will help you control your weight over the long term. For example, did you know that foods that are labeled an "excellent source" of a particular nutrient provide 20% or more of the Recommended Daily Value. Whereas, foods that are a "good source" of a nutrient provide between 10 and 20% of the Recommended Daily Value.

<h1 style="text-align:center">Day 22 - Recipe</h1>

<u>Shrimp & Spinach Salad</u>

2 pounds shrimp in shell
½ pound small green beans, trimmed
½ pound baby spinach leaves
2 tablespoon lemon juice
¼ cup extra-virgin olive oil
2 teaspoon minced fresh dill
1 tablespoon minced green onion
To make vinaigrette, combine lemon juice, olive oil, dill, salt and black pepper to taste and whisk until blended. Stir in minced onion and set aside. Steam green beans and set aside.

Peel, de-vein and butterfly shrimp. Place shrimp in a bowl and add water to cover. Add 1 teaspoon of salt, and let stand for 10 minutes. Drain, rinse, drain again, and dry. Arrange shrimp in broiling pan without a rack. Brush shrimp with a little of the vinaigrette and place under preheated broiler, about 3 inches from heat. Broil about 3 to 4 minutes, turning shrimp once, or until both sides turn pink.

Remove shrimp from broiler and add remaining vinaigrette and green beans to the broiling pan. Stir to coat shrimp and beans with vinaigrette. Pour warm vinaigrette over spinach and toss quickly. Plate the spinach and arrange shrimp and green beans on top.
<u>Serves 4</u>. 310 Calories per serving.

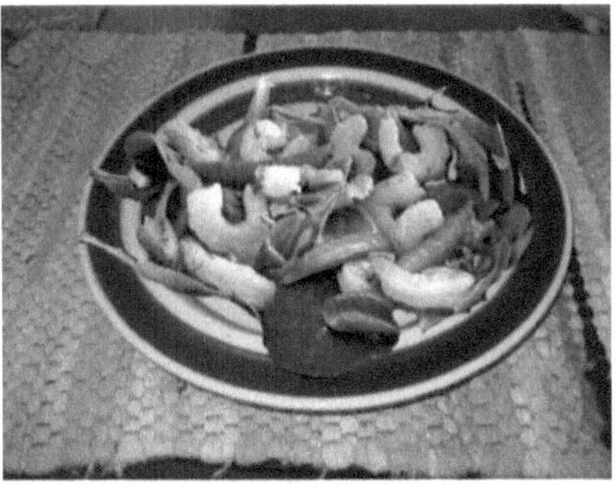

<u>Diet Tip of the Day:</u> After company leaves, have them take some of the leftover food (particularly the dessert) with them – or take the leftovers to work the next day.

Day 23 - Recipe

<u>Beans & Greens Salad</u>

   ⅓ cup chopped oregano
   ⅓ cup chopped parsley
   3 cloves garlic, chopped
   1 lemon, juiced

Prepare dressing by combining above ingredients and stirring in ¼ cup extra-virgin olive oil. Salt and black pepper to taste.

   ½ pound mesclun mix
   ¼ pound green beans
   19-oz can garbanzo beans (chickpeas)

Arrange mesclun mix, garbanzo beans and green beans on large platter. Drizzle dressing over beans and greens.

<u>Serves 4</u>. Approximately 260 Calories per serving.

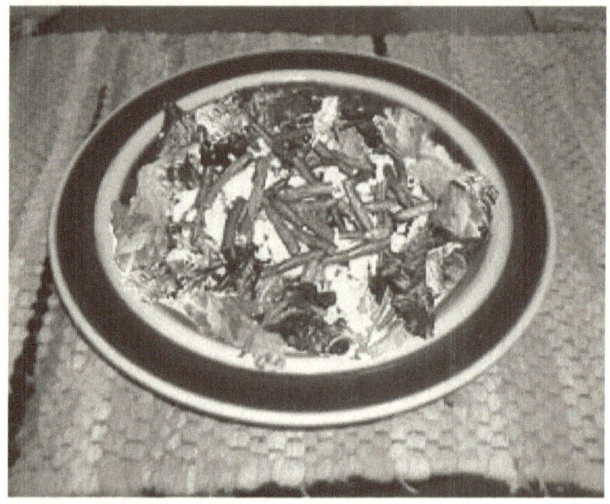

<u>Diet Tip of the Day:</u> Beans are a wonderful food but **beans are an incomplete protein**. If however beans are eaten with a whole-grain bread, the combination forms a complete protein – just as complete and nutritious as meat, poultry, or fish.

<h1 align="center">Day 24- Recipe</h1>

<u>**Four-Bean Plus Salad**</u> (This is a side dish)

Note that the total caloric value of the salad will change very little, if the proportions of the bean varieties and corn are varied – according to taste.

½ cup canned red kidney beans, drained and rinsed

½ cup canned black beans, drained and rinsed

½ cup canned chick peas, drained and rinsed

½ cup canned cannelloni beans, drained and rinsed

½ cup canned corn, drained

1 small red pepper, chopped

1 small green pepper, chopped

2 tablespoons extra-virgin olive oil

2 tablespoons lemon juice

In a large bowl mix red kidney beans, black beans, chick peas, cannelloni beans, corn and chopped red and green peppers. Stir in olive oil and lemon juice and plate.

<u>**Serves about 6**</u>. One serving is ½ cup – with about 135 Calories per serving

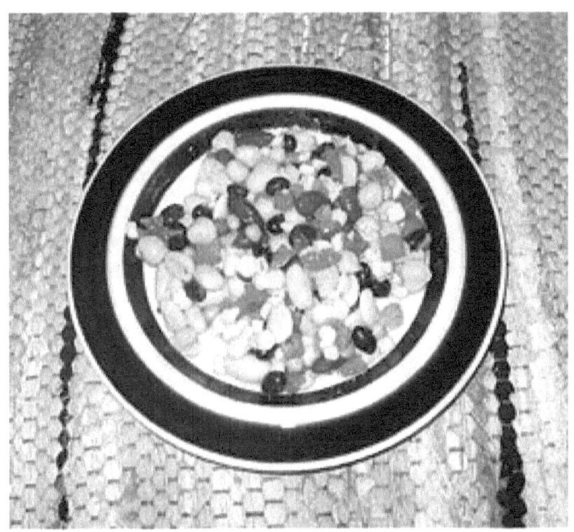

<u>**Diet Tip of the Day:**</u> Vigorous exercise doesn't necessarily stimulate you to overeat. Just the opposite. In many cases, exercise actually helps curb your appetite – immediately following a workout.

<h1 style="text-align:center">Day 25 - Recipe</h1>

<u>Pan-Broiled Hanger Steak</u>

    1¼ pounds hanger steak, well trimmed of fat
    ¼ cup lime juice
    8 small new potatoes, peeled and halved
    ½ pint cherry tomatoes (about 15), halved

Season both sides of steak with salt and pepper and place in sealable plastic bag with lime juice. Refrigerate for about one hour.

Boil potatoes about 10 minutes. Rinse in cold water. Sauté potatoes in small amount of vegetable oil over medium-high heat until brown.

Sauté cherry tomatoes in small amount of olive oil over medium-high heat until skin begins to crack. Season with chopped fresh basil.

Heat a skillet over medium-high heat. Sear hanger steak on one side for about 5 minutes. Turn over and sear other side approximately 5 minutes (for medium done). Pour off any fat that may have accumulated. Cut into ½-inch slices.

<u>Serves 4.</u> About 320 Calories per serving (for the hanger steak only)

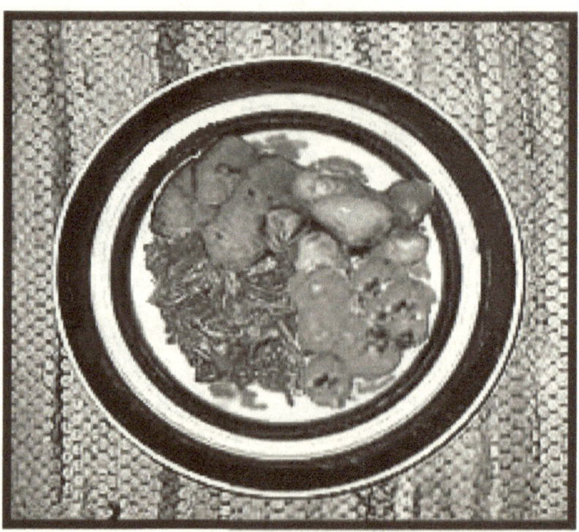

<u>Diet Tip of the Day:</u> If you go to a **party**, don't stand near the food! Be aware of the temptation. Make the effort, and you'll find you eat less.

Day 26 - Recipe
Tina's Grilled Scallops &Polenta

1 pound sea scallops
¾ cup polenta cornmeal
¾ cup skim milk
1 medium portobello mushroom
½ pound green beans
¼ cup chopped red onion
16 asparagus spear
1 teaspoon extra-virgin olive oil

Bring 1½ cups of water and skim milk to rapid boil. Add salt to taste and slowly add polenta while stirring. Reduce heat. Continue stirring until desired consistency is reached. Pour polenta into lightly greased pan. After polenta has cooled cover and refrigerate. Cut chilled polenta into 4 pieces. Grill on medium-hot fire – about two minutes on each side.

Brush portobello mushroom and asparagus spear with olive oil and place on grill for about 3 minutes on each side.

Grill scallops on medium-hot fire. Turn after two minutes or when first side turns opaque. Grill until second side turns opaque – about another 2 minutes. Don't overcook but test a scallop by cutting to make sure it's cooked through. Salt and pepper to taste.
Serves 4. The food on the plate pictured below totals about 380 Calories.

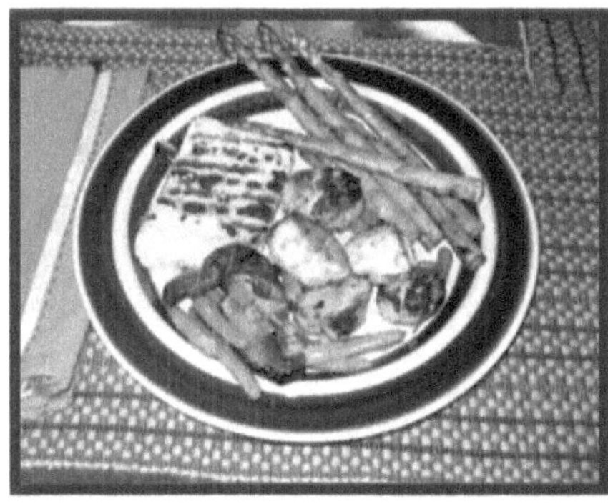

Diet Tip of the Day: To have better control of what you eat **bring your lunch to work**.

Fettuccine in Summer Sauce

This sauce is often served in the summer because it's lighter than what is usually dished up with pasta. But despite its name the sauce is wonderful year round.

    ½ lb fettuccine
    8 oz fresh asparagus, trimmed & cut in 2-inch pieces
    ¾ pint cherry tomatoes (about 20), halved
    2 Tbsp plus 1 tsp extra-virgin olive oil, divided
    2 cloves of garlic, chopped
    ½ small onion, diced

Cook fettuccine according to package directions. Drain and return pasta to pot; add a teaspoon of the olive oil and toss to coat. Meanwhile steam asparagus and drain.

In large skillet over medium-high heat, sauté cherry tomatoes in remaining 2 tablespoons of olive oil until skin begins to crack. Add onion and cook until translucent. Stir in garlic. Thin sauce with pasta liquid to desired consistency. Toss cooked pasta and asparagus into sauce and serve immediately.

Serves 4. About 290 Calories per serving

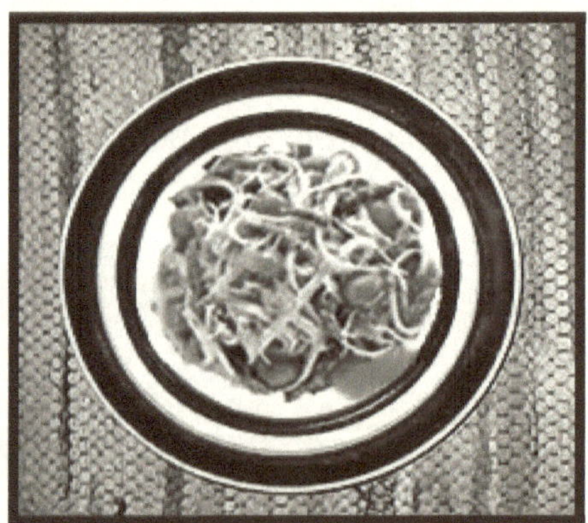

Diet Tip of the Day: A major weight-loss fallacy is that you can **get rid of abdominal fat** by working your abdominal muscles. This is based on the incorrect belief that fat is eliminated from a particular part of your body if you engage the muscles underneath that layer of fat. No such luck.

Day 28 - Recipe

<u>Frozen Chicken Dinner</u>

No recipe today. No cooking today. Another day off! There are plenty of frozen chicken choices in your local supermarket. Here are some reasonably good selections:

Crustless Chicken Pot Pie	**Smart Ones**	~~200~~ 190
Buffalo Style Chicken	**Lean Cuisine**	~~200~~ 190
Home Style Chicken & Potatoes	**Healthy Choice**	200
Honey Balsamic Chicken	**Healthy Choice**	210
Sesame Stir Fry with Chicken	**Lean Cuisine**	280
Roasted Turkey Breast	**Lean Cuisine**	~~280~~ 290
Apple Cranberry Chicken	**Lean Cuisine**	280
Chicken Fettuccini Alfredo	**Healthy Choice**	280
Grilled Chicken Marinara	**Healthy Choice**	280
Sweet & Spicy Orange Chicken	**Healthy Choice**	280
Chicken Parmesan	**Smart Ones**	280
Turkey Breast with Stuffing	**Smart Ones**	280

If you fall short of the **300 Calories allocated for today's frozen meal**. In this case, use the remaining 100 or so calories anyway you wish. Splurge on extra dessert or save the calories for another day.

See **Appendix B** on page 198 for our comprehensive list of frozen entrees. Please read the important **Frozen-Food Safety Warning** in **Appendix C** on page 203.

Day 29 - Recipe

<u>Barbequed Shrimp & Corn</u>

 1½ pounds large shrimp, peeled and de-veined
 3 Tbsp of your favorite bottled barbeque sauce
 4 medium ears of corn

Pour barbeque sauce into shallow bowl. Toss shrimp in barbeque sauce to coat. Place shrimp on medium-hot grill. Turn shrimp after about two minutes or when shrimp turn pink. Grill until second side turns pink – approximately another 2 minutes. Don't overcook but test a shrimp by cutting to make sure it is cooked through. Salt and pepper to taste. Serve hot or at room temperature.

<u>Serves 4</u>. About 160 Calories per serving (shrimp only).

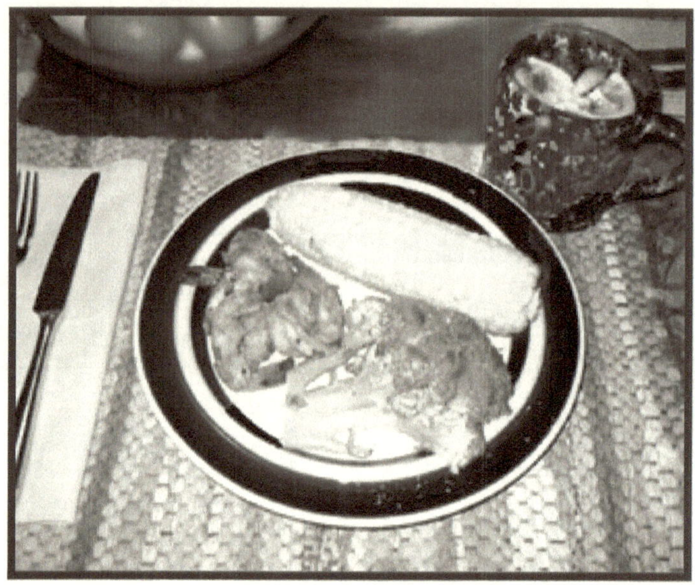

<u>Diet Tip of the Day:</u> A very **important weight-profile parameter** is your waist-to-hip ratio. Health risks for heart attack and stroke increase considerably for men with a ratio above 1.0 and for women with a ratio above 0.8. To calculate your ratio, measure your waist size (at its narrowest circumference) and divide it by your hip size (at the widest section).

Day 30 - Recipe

<u>Cheeseburger Heaven</u>

There's really not much to grilling hamburgers. The ideal meat for a
juicy burger is ground chuck with about 20% fat, but we are talking
diet here. So we opt for leaner, much leaner meat.
1¼ pounds ground sirloin (95% lean)
4 thin slices low-fat American cheese
Mix ground beef in large bowl. Salt and pepper to taste. Divide into 4
equal portions and form burgers about 1-inch thick.

Cook burgers over a hot fire on charcoal or gas-fired grill. For
medium, cook about 4 minutes on each side. Top with slice of cheese.
Add lettuce and tomato. Season to taste.

<u>Serves 4</u>. About 370 Calories per serving (cheeseburger only).

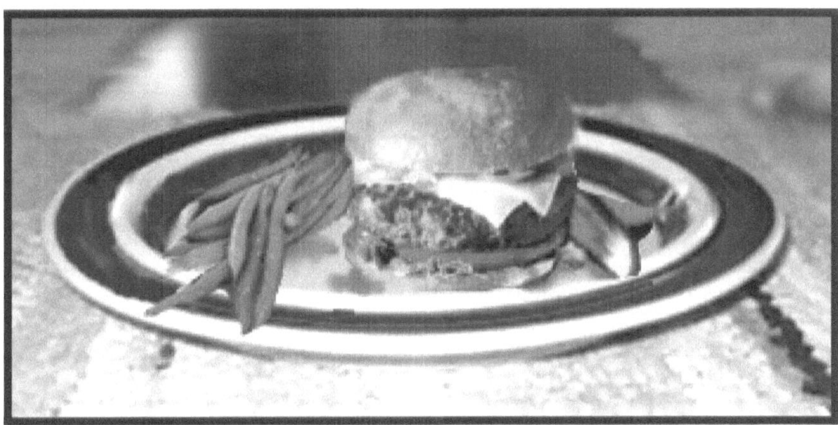

<u>Diet Tip of the Day:</u> **Plan to be on a diet the rest of your life**. Not
necessarily a weight-reducing diet. At some point you'll want to just
maintain your weight. But you will still need to continue to make good
healthy food choices – and not slip back to your old eating habits.

Appendix A
Soup Selections

When the Daily Meal Plan menu specifies soup have only one serving (8 ounces) unless stated otherwise. Note that the listed soups were available in most supermarkets as of 07/21/2020.   *These are a canned soup selections.

Soup Description	Calories
Healthy Choice Chicken with Rice	90
Campbell's Tomato	100
Healthy Choice Country Vegetable	100
Progresso Minestrone*	110
Progresso Chickarina*	110
Progresso Italian-Style Wedding*	120
Campbell's Home-Style Lite Chicken Corn Chowder*	120
Campbell's Home-Style Chicken Noodle	130
Campbell's Home-Style Butter Nut Squash*	130
Campbell's Healthy Request Vegetable Beef	140
Progresso Lentil*	140
Progresso Green Split Pea*	150
Campbell's Slow Kettle New England Clam Chowder	160
Progresso Macaroni and Bean*	160
Progresso New England Clam Chowder*	170
Progresso Lasagna-Style*	170
Progresso Broccoli Cheese with Bacon*	180
Have 2 servings of 90 Calorie soup	180
Campbell's Chunky Classic Chicken Noodle	190
Amy's Rustic Italian Vegetable*	190
Campbell's Chunky Beef n Cheese*	200
Amy's French Country Vegetable*	210
Campbell's Chunky Sirloin Burger + Vegetables	220
Enjoy two servings of a 110 or 120 Calorie soup	230
Enjoy two servings of a 120 Calorie soup	240

Appendix B
Frozen Entrees

Appendix D lists three popular brands of frozen entrées: Healthy Choice, Lean Cuisine and Smart Ones. Note that each brand is color coded. The listing is further divided by entrée type: Poultry entrées, Meat entrées, Seafood entrées, Pasta entrées, Pizza and Other entrées. The entire table is arranged from the lowest to highest in calories. Note that the listed frozen entrées were available as of 08/14/2020.

Type	Name	Brand	Calorie
Poultry	Tomato Basil Chicken & Spinach	Smart Ones	160
Meat	Steak Portobella	Lean Cuisine	160
Meat	Asian Style Beef & Broccoli	Smart Ones	170
Poultry	Herb Roasted Chicken	Lean Cuisine	170
Poultry	Slow Roasted Turkey Breast	Smart Ones	170
Poultry	Creamy Basil Chicken w Broccoli	Smart Ones	170
Poultry	Grilled Chicken Marsala	Healthy Choice	180
Poultry	Garlic Chicken Rolls	Lean Cuisine	180
Meat	Beef Merlot	Healthy Choice	180
Meat	Homestyle Beef Pot Roast	Smart Ones	180
Poultry	Roasted Turkey & Vegetables	Lean Cuisine	190
Poultry	Chicken & Broccoli Alfredo	Healthy Choice	190
Poultry	Chicken & Vegetable Stir Fry	Healthy Choice	190
Other	Broccoli & Cheddar Roast Potato	Smart Ones	190
Poultry	Crustless Chicken Pot Pie	Smart Ones	190
Poultry	Buffalo Style Chicken	Lean Cuisine	190
Poultry	Home Style Chicken & Potatoes	Healthy Choice	200
Pasta	Angel Hair Marinara	Smart Ones	200
Poultry	Salisbury Steak	Smart Ones	200
Meat	Roast Beef & Mashed Potatoes	Smart Ones	200
Pasta	Primavera Pasta	Smart Ones	210

Pasta	Ravioli Florentine	Smart Ones	210
Poultry	Cajun Style Chicken & Shrimp	Healthy Choice	220
Pasta	Cheese Ravioli Mushroom Sauce	Smart Ones	230
Poultry	Ranchero Chicken Wrap	Smart Ones	230
Poultry	Lemon Herb Chicken Picante	Smart Ones	230
Pasta	Cheese Ravioli Mushroom Sauce	Smart Ones	230
Meat	Meat Loaf with Mashed Potatoes	Lean Cuisine	240
Seafood	Shrimp Alfredo	Lean Cuisine	240
Poultry	Chicken Margherita	Smart Ones	240
Poultry	Grilled Chicken Caesar	Lean Cuisine	240
Poultry	Honey Glazed Turkey & Potatoes	Healthy Choice	240
Pasta	Spicy Penne Arrabiata	Lean Cuisine	240
Pasta	Four Cheese Cannelloni	Lean Cuisine	250
Poultry	Creamy Basil Chicken w Tortellini	Lean Cuisine	250
Pasta	Cheese Ravioli	Lean Cuisine	250
Pasta	Vermont Cheddar Mac & Cheese	Lean Cuisine	250
Pasta	Fettuccini Alfredo	Smart Ones	250
Poultry	Oriental Chicken	Smart Ones	250
Poultry	Fiesta Grilled Chicken	Lean Cuisine	250
Pasta	Chicken Linguini Red Pepper	Healthy Choice	250
Poultry	Golden Roasted Turkey Breast	Healthy Choice	250
Poultry	Chicken Mesquite	Smart Ones	250
Poultry	Chicken Oriental	Smart Ones	250
Poultry	Orange Sesame Chicken	Smart Ones	250
Poultry	Baked Chicken	Lean Cuisine	260
Poultry	Teriyaki Chicken & Vegetables	Smart Ones	260
Seafood	Tuna Noodle Casserole	Smart Ones	260
Pasta	Spaghetti with Meatballs	Lean Cuisine	260
Poultry	Creamy Chicken & Noodles	Healthy Choice	260
Meat	Barbecue Steak w Red Potatoes	Healthy Choice	260

Pasta	Creamy Rigatoni with Chicken	Smart Ones	260
Pasta	Macaroni & Cheese	Smart Ones	260
Pasta	Butternut Squash Ravioli	Lean Cuisine	260
Other	Santa Fe Rice & Beans	Smart Ones	260
Other	Coconut Chickpea Curry	Lean Cuisine	260
Poultry	Glazed Turkey Tenderloins	Lean Cuisine	270
Poultry	Kung Pao Chicken	Healthy Choice	270
Poultry	Chicken Margherita w Balsamic	Healthy Choice	270
Poultry	Chicken Strips & Sweet Potatoes	Smart Ones	270
Pasta	Sesame Noodles with Vegetables	Smart Ones	280
Pasta	Spaghetti with Meat Sauce	Smart Ones	280
Meat	Salisbury Steak w Mac & Cheese	Lean Cuisine	290
Pasta	Penne Rosa	Lean Cuisine	270
Poultry	Turkey Breast & Stuffing	Smart Ones	280
Pasta	Classic Macaroni & Beef	Lean Cuisine	270
Pasta	Mushroom Mezzaluna Ravioli	Lean Cuisine	270
Other	Asian Pot Stickers	Lean Cuisine	280
Poultry	Sesame Stir Fry w Chicken	Lean Cuisine	280
Poultry	Apple Cranberry Chicken	Lean Cuisine	280
Poultry	Chicken Fettuccini Alfredo	Healthy Choice	280
Poultry	Grilled Chicken Marinara	Healthy Choice	280
Poultry	Sweet & Spicy Orange Chicken	Healthy Choice	280
Poultry	Chicken Parmesan	Smart Ones	280
Poultry	Turkey Breast w Stuffing	Smart Ones	280
Meat	Beef & Broccoli	Healthy Choice	280
Meat	Meatball Marinara	Healthy Choice	280
Meat	Beef Teriyaki	Healthy Choice	280
Pasta	Spinach Artichoke Ravioli	Lean Cuisine	280
Other	Vegetable Fried Rice	Smart Ones	280
Pasta	Spinach Artichoke Ravioli	Lean Cuisine	280

Pasta	Linguini with Ricotta & Spinach	Lean Cuisine	280
Poultry	Chicken Fettuccini	Lean Cuisine	280
Pasta	Spaghetti & Meatballs	Healthy Choice	280
Pasta	Spaghetti with Meat Sauce	Smart Ones	280
Other	Vegetable Fried Rice	Smart Ones	280
Other	Asian Pot Stickers	Lean Cuisine	280
Poultry	Chicken with Almonds	Lean Cuisine	290
Poultry	Chicken w Peanut Sauce	Lean Cuisine	290
Seafood	Shrimp & Angel Hair Pasta	Lean Cuisine	290
Poultry	Grilled Chicken Pesto w Veggies	Healthy Choice	290
Pasta	Pasta w Swedish Meatballs	Smart Ones	290
Poultry	Roasted Turkey Breast	Lean Cuisine	290
Poultry	General Tso's Spicy Chicken	Healthy Choice	290
Poultry	Pineapple Chicken	Healthy Choice	290
Poultry	Chicken Enchiladas Suiza	Smart Ones	290
Meat	Swedish Meatballs	Lean Cuisine	290
Seafood	Lemon Pepper Fish	Healthy Choice	290
Other	Santa Fe Rice & Beans	Smart Ones	290
Pizza	Thin Crust Cheese Pizza	Smart Ones	290
Seafood	Parmesan Crusted Fish	Lean Cuisine	300
Pasta	Santa Fe-Style Rice & Beans	Lean Cuisine	300
Poultry	Roasted Turkey & Vegetables	Lean Cuisine	300
Poultry	Sweet & Sour Chicken	Lean Cuisine	300
Poultry	Crustless Chicken Pot Pie	Healthy Choice	300
Poultry	Sweet Sesame Chicken	Healthy Choice	300
Poultry	Chicken Fettuccini	Smart Ones	300
Poultry	General Tso's Chicken	Smart Ones	300
Meat	Classic Meat Loaf	Healthy Choice	300
Seafood	Tortilla Crusted Fish	Lean Cuisine	310
Pasta	Tuscan-Style Vegetable Lasagna	Lean Cuisine	310

Pasta	Tortellini w Red Pepper Sauce	Lean Cuisine	310
Pasta	Broccoli Cheddar Rotini	Lean Cuisine	300
Pasta	Three Cheese Ziti Marinara	Smart Ones	300
Pasta	Lasagna Florentine	Smart Ones	300
Seafood	Tortilla Crusted Fish	Lean Cuisine	310
Pasta	Tuscan-Style Vegetable Lasagna	Lean Cuisine	310
Poultry	Chicken Fried Rice	Lean Cuisine	310
Poultry	Orange Chicken	Lean Cuisine	310
Poultry	Chicken Tikka Masala	Lean Cuisine	310
Poultry	Chicken Strips & Fries	Smart Ones	310
Poultry	Chicken Teriyaki	Lean Cuisine	310
Pizza	Thin Crust Pepperoni Pizza	Smart Ones	310
Pasta	Three Cheese Macaroni	Smart Ones	310
Pizza	French Bread Pepperoni Pizza	Lean Cuisine	310
Poultry	Chicken Spinach Mushroom Panini	Lean Cuisine	310
Other	Spicy Beef & Bean Enchilada	Lean Cuisine	310
Poultry	Chicken Fried Rice	Healthy Choice	320
Meat	Sweet & Spicy Korean Beef	Lean Cuisine	320
Pizza	Farmers Market Pizza	Lean Cuisine	320
Pizza	Margherita Pizza	Lean Cuisine	320
Poultry	Chicken Carbonara	Lean Cuisine	330
Poultry	Mango Chicken w Coconut Rice	Lean Cuisine	330
Poultry	Country Fried Chicken	Healthy Choice	330
Other	Cheese & Fire-Roasted Tamale	Lean Cuisine	330
Poultry	Chicken Club Panini	Lean Cuisine	340
Meat	Philly Style Steak & Cheese Panini	Lean Cuisine	350
Poultry	Chicken Parmigiana	Healthy Choice	360
Poultry	Chicken Pecan	Lean Cuisine	370
Poultry	Sweet & Sour Chicken	Healthy Choice	390
Pizza	Supreme Pizza	Lean Cuisine	390

Increasingly, food giants like ConAgra, Nestlé and others that supply Americans with processed foods concede that they cannot ensure the safety of their food products. Frozen foods pose a particularly serious safety problem because unsuspecting consumers buy frozen foods for their convenience and incorrectly believe that cooking frozen foods is a matter of taste – not safety.

Still the food industry says that extensive outbreaks of food-borne illness are rare, even though it is well-known that most of the millions of cases of food-borne illness every year go unreported or are not traced to the source. For example, each year approximately 40,000 cases of salmonella poisoning are reported in the United States – but perhaps as many as one million cases go unreported. How could this happen? First, the supply chain for ingredients in processed foods – from flour to fruits and vegetables to flavorings – is becoming more complex and global in the drive to keep food costs down. As a result, government and industry officials concede that almost every food ingredient is now a potential carrier of pathogens. A further complication is that a large number of food companies subcontract processing work to save money and don't require suppliers to test for pathogens. In fact, companies often don't even know who is supplying their ingredients.

In addition, many frozen-food manufacturers have stopped cooking their products at high temperatures, a tactic they call the "kill step," which is intended to eliminate any lingering microbes. Frequently this process step turns some of the frozen food ingredients into mush. So, instead the "kill step" has been shifted to consumers. For example, ConAgra has added food safety instructions to its frozen meals, including the Healthy Choice brand. A typical "frozen-food safety" instruction offers this guidance: "Internal temperature needs to reach 165°F as measured by a food thermometer in several spots."

Moreover, General Mills, now advises consumers to avoid microwaves altogether and cook their frozen pizzas only in a conventional oven. **<u>Bottom line</u>**: To be safe, always cook frozen foods so that the internal temperature reaches 165°F as measured by a good food thermometer.

A convenient way to determine what you should weigh is to use our New BMI-Based Weight vs. Height Chart shown in the following table, where normal weight corresponds to a BMI = 18.6 to 24.9, overweight is for BMI = 25.0 to 29.9 and obese is for BMI = 30.0 to 39.9.

Admittedly the weights in the following table would be difficult for most senior women to achieve. But consider the weights shown to be a goal.

Height	Normal	Overweight	Obese
4' 10"	90 – 119	120 – 142	143 – 191
4' 11"	93 – 123	124 – 148	149 – 197
5' 0"	96 – 127	128 – 152	153 – 204
5' 1"	99 – 131	132 – 158	159 – 211
5' 2"	102 – 135	136 – 163	164 – 218
5' 3"	105 – 140	141 – 169	170 – 225
5' 4"	109 – 144	145 – 173	174 – 232
5' 5"	112 – 149	150 – 180	181 – 239
5' 6"	116 – 154	155 – 185	186 – 247
5' 7"	119 – 159	160 – 191	192 – 254
5' 8"	123 – 163	164 – 196	197 – 262
5' 9"	126 – 168	169 – 202	203 – 270
5' 10"	130 – 173	174 – 206	207 – 278
5' 11"	134 – 178	179 – 214	215 – 286
6' 0"	137 – 183	184 – 220	221 – 294
6' 1"	141 – 188	189 – 227	228 – 302
6' 2"	145 – 194	195 – 232	233 – 310
6' 3"	149 – 199	200 – 239	240 – 319
6' 4"	152 – 205	206 - 246	247 - 328
6' 5"	157 - 210	211 - 252	253 – 337
6' 6"	161 - 216	217 - 259	260 - 346

Appendix E
Weight Loss Predction
For Senior Women

Weight loss occurs when your food energy intake is less than the total energy you expend. This difference in calories is referred to as your calorie deficit. How much weight you lose depends on the magnitude of your calorie deficit. Physiologists have long known that to lose one pound requires a deficit of approximately 3,500 Calories. Therefore, if a person's total calorie deficit over time is known, their weight loss over time can be calculated. Fortunately, a more precise determination of the rate of weight loss is possible. Scientists have demonstrated that **weight loss is a function of age, sex, height, weight, physical activity, caloric intake and the duration of the diet (or time on the diet)**. This writer related all these variables in a complex, scientifically based, energy-weight-control equation, published in the *American Journal of Clinical Nutrition,,* and subsequently published a set of 60 Weight Loss Prediction tables in the paperback *The Computer Diet* (now published by NoPaperPress). In this book you will find an abridged set of six Weight Loss Prediction tables specifically for senior women.

Selecting the Correct Table
Your first task is to choose the correct Weight Loss Prediction Table. The six Weight Loss Prediction Tables are organized by gender, age and activity level. The three activity levels most applicable to seniors are covered in this text:

1) Sedentary: Inactive most of the day with very little standing or walking.

2) Relatively Inactive: Seated most of the day with about four hours of standing and incidental walking.

3) Moderately Active: To qualify for this category, you have to engage in some form of regular exercise everyday (e.g., taking a brisk three-mile walk).

Use the following table to find the Weight Loss Prediction Table that is applicable to you.

Gender	Age	Activity Level	Table/Page
Women	50 - 65	Sedentary	**E1/86**
	50 - 65	Inactive	**E2/87**
	50 - 65	Active	**E3/88**
	66 - 80	Sedentary	**E4/89**
	66 - 80	Inactive	**E5/90**
	66 - 80	Active	**E6/91**

Weight Loss Prediction Tables

Weight Loss Prediction Example

Consider a 63-year-old woman, who is 5' 2" and 160 pounds, is retired does some light house work but spends most of her free time watching TV. How long will it take her to lose 20 pounds?

First from the above list of tables, she should choose **Table E2** labeled "Weight Loss Prediction for Relatively Inactive Women, Ages 50 - 65 years." Then she would scan the far left of the table and locate her present weight of 160 pounds; from this number she would run a finger horizontally (to the right) until it intersects the vertical column headed by the 20-pound weight loss she desires. The three numbers at the intersection are the time in days to lose 20 pounds, depending on the diet calories consumed. Specifically, to lose 20 pounds our fictional female's diet calorie options are:

- 900 Cal per day for 59 days.
- 1200 Cal per day for 76 days.
- 1500 Cal per day for 107 days.

Which alternative should she choose? Health professionals recommend a gradual weight loss of one to two pounds per week. In this case, that would mean her diet should last 10 to 20 weeks or 70 to 140 days, pointing to the 1200-Calorie diet option. Let's assume our fictional dieter decides on 1200 Calories. The above suggests that it will take her about 76 days to lose 20 pounds.

Incidentally, most senior women are not quite satisfied but are usually not hungry on a 1200-Calorie diet. In addition a 1200-Calorie diet provides substantial weight loss. For these reasons this book presents only 1200 Calorie diets with Daily Menus.

Table E1: Weight Loss for Sedentary Women - 51 to 65

Present Weight	Diet Calories	Weight Loss (lbs)							
		5	10	15	20	30	40	50	60
120 lbs	900	21	42			Numbers in table indicate time in days to lose weight.			
	1200	30	63						
	1500	57	123						
130 lbs	900	19	39	59	81				
	1200	27	55	85	118				
	1500	45	96	153	219				
140 lbs	900	17	36	54	74	117			
	1200	24	49	76	104	167			
	1500	38	79	124	174	298			
160 lbs	900	15	31	47	64	99	138		
	1200	20	40	62	85	134	189		
	1500	28	59	91	126	204	300		
180 lbs	900	13	27	41	56	87	120	155	
	1200	17	35	53	72	112	156	205	
	1500	23	47	72	99	158	225	304	
200 lbs	900	12	25	37	50	78	107	137	170
	1200	15	30	46	63	97	134	175	219
	1500	19	40	61	82	130	182	240	307
220 lbs	1200	11	22	34	46	70	96	123	152
	1500	13	27	41	56	86	118	153	190
	1800	16	34	52	71	110	153	200	253
240 lbs	1200	10	21	31	42	64	88	112	138
	1500	12	25	37	50	77	106	136	168
	1800	15	30	46	62	96	133	173	216

Table E2: Weight Loss Relatively Inactive Women- 51 to 65

Present Weight	Diet Calories	Weight Loss (lbs)							
		5	10	15	20	30	40	50	60
120 lbs	900	19	39			Numbers in table indicate time in days to lose weight.			
	1200	27	56						
	1500	46	98						
130 lbs	900	17	35	54	74				
	1200	24	49	76	105				
	1500	37	79	124	176				
140 lbs	900	16	33	50	68	107			
	1200	21	44	67	93	148			
	1500	32	66	103	144	242			
160 lbs	900	14	28	43	59	91	127		
	1200	18	36	56	76	119	168		
	1500	20	50	78	107	173	252		
180 lbs	900	12	25	38	52	80	110	143	
	1200	15	31	47	65	101	140	184	
	1500	20	41	63	86	136	193	259	
200 lbs	900	11	23	34	46	71	98	126	157
	1200	13	27	42	56	87	121	157	197
	1500	17	35	53	72	113	158	208	265
220 lbs	1200	10	21	31	42	65	88	113	140
	1500	12	24	37	50	78	107	138	171
	1800	15	30	46	62	97	134	175	220
240 lbs	1200	9	19	29	39	59	81	103	127
	1500	11	22	34	45	70	96	123	152
	1800	13	27	41	55	85	117	152	190

Table E3: Weight Loss for Moderately Active Women 51 to 65

Present Weight	Diet Calories	Weight Loss (lbs)							
		5	10	15	20	30	40	50	60
120 lbs	900	16	33			Numbers in table indicate time in days to lose weight.			
	1200	21	44						
	1500	32	67						
130 lbs	900	15	30	46	63				
	1200	19	39	60	83				
	1500	27	56	88	123				
140 lbs	900	14	28	42	58	91			
	1200	17	35	54	74	118			
	1500	23	48	75	104	171			
160 lbs	900	12	24	37	50	77	107		
	1200	14	29	45	62	97	136		
	1500	19	38	59	81	129	185		
180 lbs	900	10	21	32	44	68	94	121	
	1200	13	25	39	53	82	114	149	
	1500	15	32	49	66	104	147	195	
200 lbs	900	9	19	29	39	61	83	107	133
	1200	11	22	34	46	72	99	128	160
	1500	13	27	41	56	88	123	161	203
220 lbs	1200	9	17	26	36	55	75	96	119
	1500	10	20	31	41	64	88	113	140
	1800	12	24	36	49	76	106	137	172
240 lbs	1200	8	16	24	33	50	67	87	108
	1500	9	18	28	37	58	79	101	125
	1800	10	21	32	44	68	93	120	149

Table E4: Weight Loss for Sedentary Women - 66 to 80

Present Weight	Diet Calories	Weight Loss (lbs)							
		5	10	15	20	30	40	50	60
120 lbs	900	22	46						
	1200	34	72			Numbers in table indicate time in days to lose weight.			
	1500	73	161						
130 lbs	900	20	42	64	88				
	1200	30	62	96	133				
	1500	55	118	191	279				
140 lbs	900	19	38	59	80	126			
	1200	26	54	84	116	188			
	1500	44	94	149	212				
160 lbs	900	16	33	50	68	107	148		
	1200	22	44	68	93	147	209		
	1500	32	67	104	145	239	357		
180 lbs	900	14	29	44	60	93	128	167	
	1200	18	37	57	78	122	171	225	
	1500	26	53	81	112	179	257	350	
200 lbs	900	13	26	40	54	83	113	146	282
	1200	16	33	50	67	105	145	190	238
	1500	21	43	67	91	144	203	271	348
220 lbs	1200	12	24	36	48	75	102	131	162
	1500	14	29	44	60	92	127	165	205
	1800	18	37	57	78	121	169	221	280
240 lbs	1200	11	22	32	44	67	93	119	146
	1500	13	26	40	54	83	113	146	181
	1800	16	33	50	68	105	145	189	236

Table E5: Weight Loss Relatively Inactive Women- 66 to 80

Present Weight	Diet Calories	Weight Loss (lbs)							
		5	10	15	20	30	40	50	60
120 lbs	900	20	42						
	1200	31	62			Numbers in table indicate time in days to lose weight.			
	1500	56	120						
130 lbs	900	19	38	59	80				
	1200	26	54	84	116				
	1500	44	93	148	213				
140 lbs	900	17	35	54	115	162			
	1200	23	48	74	164	238			
	1500	36	76	120	289				
160 lbs	900	15	30	46	62	97	136		
	1200	19	39	60	82	130	184		
	1500	27	56	87	121	197	290		
180 lbs	900	13	27	40	55	85	117	152	190
	1200	16	33	51	70	109	152	200	254
	1500	22	45	95	95	151	216	292	
200 lbs	900	12	24	36	49	76	104	134	166
	1200	14	29	45	60	94	130	169	212
	1500	18	38	58	79	124	174	230	295
220 lbs	1200	11	22	33	43	68	93	120	148
	1500	13	26	40	54	83	114	147	183
	1800	16	33	50	67	105	146	191	241
240 lbs	1200	10	20	30	41	62	85	109	134
	1500	12	34	36	48	74	102	131	162
	1800	14	39	44	59	92	127	164	205

Table E6: Weight Loss for Moderately Active Women 66 to 80

Present Weight	Diet Calories	Weight Loss (lbs)							
		5	10	15	20	30	40	50	60
120 lbs	900	17	35						
	1200	23	48			Numbers in table indicate time in days to lose weight.			
	1500	36	77						
130 lbs	900	16	32	49	67				
	1200	21	42	66	90				
	1500	30	63	99	140				
140 lbs	900	14	29	45	61	96			
	1200	18	38	58	80	128			
	1500	16	54	84	117	193			
160 lbs	900	12	25	39	52	82	114		
	1200	15	31	48	66	104	146		
	1500	20	42	64	88	142	205		
180 lbs	900	11	22	34	46	71	99	128	
	1200	13	27	41	56	87	122	159	
	1500	17	34	52	72	113	160	213	
200 lbs	900	10	20	30	41	63	87	113	140
	1200	12	24	36	49	76	105	136	171
	1500	14	29	44	60	94	132	173	220
220 lbs	1200	9	18	28	37	57	78	101	124
	1500	10	21	32	43	67	92	119	148
	1800	12	25	39	52	81	113	147	184
240 lbs	1200	8	17	25	34	52	71	91	112
	1500	9	19	29	39	60	83	107	132
	1800	11	23	34	46	72	99	128	159

NoPaperPress eBooks and Paperbacks

100-Day Super Diet-1200 Cal*
100-Day Super Diet-1500 Cal*
100-Day No-Cooking Diet-1200 Cal*
100-Day No-Cooking Diet-1500 Cal*
31 Smart Diet-1200 Cal*
90-Day Smart Diet-1500 Cal*
90-Day No-Cooking Diet - 1200 Cal*
90-Day No-Cooking Diet - 1500 Cal*
90-Day Perfect Diet - 1200 Cal*
90-Day Perfect Diet - 1500 Cal*
60-Day Perfect Diet-1200 Cal*
60-Day Perfect Diet-1500 Cal*
50-Day Flex Diet-1200 Cal*
50-Day Flex Diet-1500 Cal*
30-Day Quick Diet - Women*
30-Day Quick Diet for Men*
30-Day No-Cooking Diet*
30-Day Diet for Women - Metric*
30-Day Diet for Men - Metric*
25 Day Easy Diet-1200 Cal*
25 Day Easy Diet-1500 Cal*
25-Day No-Cooking Diet
10-Day Express Diet
10-Day No-Cooking Diet*
7-Day Diet for Women*
7-Day Diet for Men*
7-Day No-Cooking Diets*
90-Day Gluten-Free Diet-1200 Cal*
90-Day Gluten-Free Diet-1500 Cal*
30-Day Gluten-Free Quick Diet*
30-Day Gluten-Free No-Cooking*
7-Day Diet for Women - Metric*
7-Day Diet for Men - Metric
7-Day Gluten-Free Express Diet*
7-Day Gluten-Free No-Cooking Diet*
90-Day Vegetarian Diet-1200 Cal*
90-Day Vegetarian Diet-1500 Cal*
30-Day Vegetarian Diet*
7-Day Vegetarian Diet*
Weight Loss for Women*
Weight Loss for Women - Metric
Weight Loss for Women - UK
Weight Loss for Men*
Maximum Weight Loss - 1200 Cal*
Maximum Weight Loss - 1500 Cal*

Weight Loss for Men - Metric*
Maximum Weight Loss- 1200 Cal*
Maximum Weight Loss- 1500 Cal*
Weight Control - U.S. Edition*
Weight Control - Metric. Edition
Prof Weight Control Women - U.S.
Prof Weight Control Women - Metric
Prof Weight Control Men - U.S.
Prof Weight Control Men - Metric
Weight Maintenance - U.S. Ed*
Weight Maintenance - Metric. Ed*
Weight Maintenance - UK Ed
Weight Loss for Senior Men*
Weight Loss for Senior Women*
Eat Smart - U.S. Edition*
Eat Smart - Metric Edition
30-Day Mediterranean Diet
Exercise Smart - U.S. Edition*
Exercise Smart - Metric Edition
Exercise Smart - UK Edition*
Total Fitness - U.S. Edition
Total Fitness - Metric Edition
Total Fitness - UK Edition
Total Fitness for Women-U.S. Ed*
Total Fitness for Women - Metric
Total Fitness for Women - UK Ed
Total Fitness for Men - U.S. Ed*
Total Fitness for Men- Metric Ed*
Total Fitness for Men - UK Ed
Senior Fitness - U.S. Edition*
Senior Fitness - Metric Edition*
Senior Fitness - UK Edition*
Computer Diet - U.S. Edition*
Computer Diet - Metric Ed*
Reliable Weight Loss - U.S. Ed
101 Weight Loss Tips*
101 Healthy Eating Tips*
101 Lifelong Fitness Tips*
101 Weight Maintenance Tips
101 Weight Loss Recipes
101 GF Weight Loss Recipes
101 Veggie Weight Loss Recipes*
30-Day Mediterranean Diet*
90-Day Mediterranean Diet - 1200 Cal*
90-Day Mediterranean Diet - 1500 Cal*

* These titles are available as both ebooks and paperbacks. Our ebooks are sold by Amazon, Apple, Google, Barnes & Noble and Kobo, but our paperbacks are only sold by Amazon.

Disclaimer

This book offers general meal planning, nutrition and weight control information. It is not a medical manual and the author does not claim to be medically qualified. The material in this book is not intended to be a substitute for medical counseling. Everyone should have a medical checkup before beginning a weight loss program. Moreover, the physician conducting the medical exam should be made aware of and should approve the specific weight control program planned. Additionally, while the author and publisher have made every effort to ensure the accuracy of the information in this book, they make no representations or warranties regarding its accuracy or completeness. Further, neither the author nor publisher assume liability for any medical problems that might result from applying the methods in this book, or for any loss of profit, or any other commercial damages, including but not limited to special, incidental, consequential or other damages, and any such liability is hereby expressly disclaimed.